PUBLIC HEALTH IN THE 21ST CENTURY

RARE DISEASES

DIAGNOSES, CHALLENGES AND DEVELOPING TREATMENTS

PUBLIC HEALTH IN THE 21ST CENTURY

Additional books in this series can be found on Nova's website
under the Series tab.

Additional e-books in this series can be found on Nova's website
under the e-book tab.

PUBLIC HEALTH IN THE 21ST CENTURY

RARE DISEASES

DIAGNOSES, CHALLENGES AND DEVELOPING TREATMENTS

GIORGIO DI GIOVANNI
AND
PIETRO MARCOZ
EDITORS

New York

Library of Congress Cataloging-in-Publication Data

ISBN: 978-1-62948-525-6

Library of Congress Control Number: 2013952594

Published by Nova Science Publishers, Inc. † New York

Contents

Preface

A rare disease is any disease that affects a small percentage of the population. Rare diseases can vary in prevalence between populations, so a disease that is rare in some populations may be common in others. This is especially true of genetic diseases and infectious diseases. In this book, the authors present current research on the diagnoses, challenges and developing treatments for rare diseases, from researchers across the globe. Topics discussed include commotio cordis, also known as cardiac concussion with described cases of ventricular fibrillation and sudden death from cardiac arrest; the clinical manifestations and pathophysiology of muscle-specific kinase (MuSK) myasthenia gravis (MG); neurological complications of histiocytosis; nail-patella syndrome; management of cardiac angiosarcoma; diagnosis and treatment of clear cell adenocarcinoma of the bladder; eosinophilic pancreatitis; non-traumatic splenic rupture; and alkaptonuria (AKU).

Chapter I – Commotio cordis, also known as concussion of the heart or cardiac concussion, is a Latin term used to describe cases of ventricular fibrillation and sudden death from cardiac arrest in a youth may occur during sports play after a blunt blow to the chest in the absence of structural cardiovascular disease or traumatic injury. It is rare, but being with increasing frequency recently. Commotio cordis was systemically described in the beginning of the 20th century by Schlomka, but the etiology of commotio cordis remained elusive until recent years. It is now apparent that commotio cordis is a mechano-electric coupling event, and it is associated with ion channels. Due to the rapid development and particularity of injury, it is a challenge to diagnose of commotio cordis. The ECG of commotio cordis is nonspecific, and the autopsy founding generally could not reveal any underlying congenital or acquired heart disease in victims. Of note, the primary treatment is another challenge for medical staff and bystanders. Likely due to a lack of early recognition and the failure to initiate timely aggressive resuscitation and defibrillation, the survival rate in the USCCR is present to be nearly 15%. Based on the epidemiological date, more widespread access to automated external defibrillator at organized youth sporting events and the training of personnel in their early use would likely achieve substantial increase in the survival of the victims. Moreover, several preventive strategies have been considered, including increasing the use of softer balls and effective chest wall protectors, but it needs to be improved in the future.

Chapter II – Rare diseases often have a negative impact on the personal, professional and social life of the patients. For this reason, taking into account both the medical and the social dimensions of the disease in patients' follow-up could improve patients' experience of the illness. However, implementing such a comprehensive approach can be difficult, because the related information, the skills or the temporal or material resources are not always available to medical teams. One way to fill this gap is to work in partnership with the associations dedicated to rare disorders. Indeed, these associations gather a large proportion of patients. Even more numerous are the patients who only temporarily join in order to address a specific problem that the medical team had not been able to address directly or precisely. Some characteristics of these associations tend to affect the relationships with the medical teams who would be willing to set up a cooperation. For this reason, it is useful to distinguish three different types of associations with respect to this potential cooperation. Finally, as there are many rare diseases, public policies targeting these conditions increasingly aim at taking an approach that address several rare diseases simultaneously. One way to develop such a global approach is to focus on the issues that are common to several rare (and to some frequent) diseases. This issue-based approach is fortunately a key feature of the work carried out in some rare disease associations, and as such, it could be useful for medical teams wishing to develop the global, cross-disease vision that public policies are asking for.

Chapter III – Muscle-specific kinase (MuSK) myasthenia gravis (MG) is a relatively rare autoimmune disease. Although it shares many features with the more common form of autoimmune myasthenia, i.e., acetylcholine receptor (AChR)-positive, there are many differences in the clinical manifestations, pathophysiology and response to treatment. This leads to significant difficulties in the diagnosis and management of this illness. Whereas the function of the AChR is well understood, this is not so regarding MuSK. Little is known about the roles of this complex protein. In the embryonic period it is essential for proper assembly of the neuromuscular junction, but emerging evidence suggests that it may have other roles as well. Conflicting data obtained from different patient groups and experimental models suggest that anti-MuSK antibodies are not uniform, and therefore exert a different effect depending on the epitope they are directed to. Furthermore, most of the data in the medical literature is based on patients who have evidence for neuromuscular transmission defects. Yet, there are sporadic descriptions and case reports which suggest that other mechanisms may be at play.

Chapter IV – Histiocytosis represents a group of rare diseases presenting with different demographic, clinical, imaging, histological and molecular characteristics. The primary molecular pathology arises in and causes proliferation of tissue macrophages or histiocytes, elements of the lymphoreticular system. The three most commonly encountered forms, Langerhans cell histiocytosis (LCH), Erdheim-Chester Disease (ECD) and Rosai-Dorfman disease (RDD), typically affect pediatric, adult, and pediatric - young adult age groups, respectively. The range and severity of organ involvements span from a single organ (e.g., cutis) disease with good prognosis to multiple, high-risk organ (e.g., heart, lung, brain, bone marrow) involvements with increased morbidity and mortality. When clinical and paraclinical data raise the suspicion for the entity, histological and immunohistochemical examination of lesions can verify the diagnosis and the actual subtype of histiocytosis. Involvement of the central nervous system (CNS) is common in each form, and is associated with significant diagnostic and treatment challenges. While evidence-based information from placebo-controlled, randomized and double-blind trials is as yet unavailable, empirical data provide useful guidance for choosing effective treatment modalities in each of these conditions. Recent studies also reveal molecular substrates of transformation from tissue residential to pathological histiocytes, highlight the importance of acquired somatic mutations in the pathogenesis and identify potential new targets for therapy.

Chapter V – Nail-patella syndrome (NPS) is an autosomal dominant disorder reported in 1/50000 individuals. It has been mapped to the long arm of chromosome 9 (9q34) with mutations in LMX1B gene. Diagnosis is usually based on clinical findings. Cardinal anomalies of NPS are dysplasia of the nails, hypoplasia or absence of the patellae, presence of iliac horns and elbow abnormalities. Additionally some patients develop glomerulopathy and primary open angle glaucoma (POAG) along with other anomalies. Progression to renal failure occurs in about 10% of NPS patients requiring either dialysis or kidney transplantation.

Chapter VI – Quality literature for management of cardiac angiosarcoma is shortly supplied due to the low incidence and its poor prognosis. A multidisciplinary management of these tumours is radically important, offering surgery or even cardiac transplant for the few potentially resectable patients. Even after complete resection, early recurrence and distant spread are the rule. Chemotherapy would be the treatment of choice for those patients diagnosed with distant metastases (56-80%) and for those with distant relapse after surgery. Most of the chemotherapy schedules employed are those with known efficacy for other soft tissue sarcoma. Nevertheless there are important characteristics in the pathology of these tumours that might have impact in the systemic treatment. As it happened with the Kaposi sarcoma, cardiac angiosarcomas are derived from endothelial cells and angiogenesis seems to be an important and druggable target. The employment of drugs with known antiangiogenic treatment like the anti-VEGF monoclonal antibody (bevacizumab) or multi-kinase inhibitors such as sorafenib and sunitib have been tested. Epidemiology, diagnosis and management of cardiac angiosarcomas will be reviewed, focusing in the available data for target therapies.

Chapter VII – Clear cell adenocarcinoma (CCA) is an extremely rare variant of adenocarcinoma of the bladder. In contrast to the common urothelial carcinoma of the bladder, CCA affects women more often than men. Since it was first reported in 1968, only a few reports have been available on this rare disease. Accurate recognition and diagnosis for clear cell adenocarcinoma of the bladder is difficult due to its rarity and uncharacteristic clinical presentation. Moreover, it is relatively more malignant with poor prognosis than the common urothelial carcinoma. Experiences are still accumulating in treating this disease. In this review, the authors characterized clinical aspects of clear cell adenocarcinoma of the bladder, including epidemiology, clinical presentation, diagnosis, treatment and prognosis. This may help the clinicians to recognize and diagnose this rare bladder carcinoma, and formulate treatment recommendations.

Chapter VIII – Eosinophilic pancreatitis (EP) is an extremely rare clinical entity. So far, only 26 cases of EP have been reported in the medical literature. Most of the patients with EP are also affected by eosinophilic gastroenteritis (EG) (88%) or idiopathic hypereosinophilic syndrome (HIS). Hypersensitivity reactions and milk allergy are considered common etiological factors for both EP and EG. For the majority of patients, the diagnosis can be challenging because of the wide array of non-specific symptoms such as recurrent abdominal pain, diarrhea and weight loss. The main treatment of EP is the use of steroids and the prognosis is usually favorable with resolution of the symptoms and histopahological findings. Endoscopy is often used to obtain biopsies and to insert temporary stents in the biliary or pancreatic ducts in patients who present with jaundice or pancreatic duct obstruction.

Chapter IX – Splenic rupture is a rare cause of abdominal pain and carries a high mortality rate. While the most common cause is trauma, it may occur due to the complications of infectious, neoplastic and hematologic diseases. Patients usually suffer from acute abdominal pain in the left upper quadrant, nausea, vomiting, and dizziness. Ultrasonography is important for diagnosis and abdominal computed tomography is important especially for staging the splenic rupture. For the treatment, either splenectomy or follow-up (especially for low-grade splenic ruptures) can be done. The therapy of choice can vary between patients depending on grade of splenic rupture, hemodynamic instability, availability of endovascular treatment and preference of the treating physician. Treatment should be focused on preserving splenic tissue. Non-traumatic rupture of the spleen must be considered by physicians in patients presenting with acute abdominal pain even without evident history of trauma, since early recognition and treatment can prevent serious morbidity and mortality. It has the same clinical picture as traumatic rupture of the spleen but the presentation can be vague and easily missed due to the absence of trauma or other predisposing factors. Increased awareness of this condition would enhance early diagnosis and effective treatment.

Chapter X – Alkaptonuria (AKU) is the world's first genetic disease. Discovered over 100 years ago, it still has no cure. For the past decade, the AKU Society has worked towards patients' dreams of finding an effective treatment. Through funding basic research, building clinical knowledge of AKU and collaborating with industry and clinical trial experts, the AKU Society is close to achieving this. The authors united their contacts into a public-private partnership, called the DevelopAKUre consortium. Together the authors raised €6 million through a European Commission Seventh Framework Programme grant with a further €4 million through co-financing. After seeking scientific advice from the European Medicines Agency (EMA), the authors launched a series of international clinical trials in November last year. They incorporate three studies: SONIA 1 (a phase II dose-ranging study), SONIA 2 (a phase III clinical efficacy study) and SOFIA (a comparison study of young and old AKU patients to assess what age is best to begin treatment). The AKU Society is leading on patient recruitment and retention and has faced many challenges converting their experiences of recruitment in the UK for a national treatment centre into recruitment throughout Europe for clinical trials. In this article, the authors discuss the difficulties in diagnosis of a rare disease, the lessons learnt from building an international consortium to launch clinical trials and the challenges in running patient recruitment on a European scale.

In: Rare Diseases
Editors: Giorgio Di Giovanni and Pietro Marcoz

ISBN: 978-1-62948-525-6

Chapter I

Commotio Cordis: A Rare Catastrophic Mechano-Electric Coupling

Na Zheng, Ming Dong and Jie Liu*
Department of pathophysiology,
Shenzhen University School of Medicine,
Guangdong, China

Abstract

Commotio cordis, also known as concussion of the heart or cardiac concussion, is a Latin term used to describe cases of ventricular fibrillation and sudden death from cardiac arrest in a youth may occur during sports play after a blunt blow to the chest in the absence of structural cardiovascular disease or traumatic injury. It is rare, but being with increasing frequency recently. Commotio cordis was systemically described in the beginning of the 20th century by Schlomka, but the etiology of commotio cordis remained elusive until recent years.

It is now apparent that commotio cordis is a mechano-electric coupling event, and it is associated with ion channels. Due to the rapid development and particularity of injury, it is a challenge to diagnose of commotio cordis. The ECG of commotio cordis is nonspecific, and the autopsy founding generally could not reveal any underlying congenital or acquired heart disease in victims. Of note, the primary treatment is another challenge for medical staff and bystanders. Likely due to a lack of early recognition and the failure to initiate timely aggressive resuscitation and defibrillation, the survival rate in the USCCR is present to be nearly 15%. Based on the epidemiological date, more widespread access to automated external defibrillator at organized youth sporting events and the training of personnel in their early use would likely achieve substantial increase in the survival of the victims. Moreover, several preventive strategies have been considered, including increasing the use of softer balls and effective chest wall protectors, but it needs to be improved in the future.

* Corresponding Author address: Nanhai Road 3688#, Shenzhen, Guangdong Province, P.R. China. Email: lvmoyang@126.com.

Keywords: Commotio cordis; sudden cardiac death; mechano-electric coupling; ventricular fibrillation; automated external defibrillator

The Definition of Commotio Cordis

Despite blunt force cardiac damage was first introduced by Rota in 1550, commotio cordis was not systemically described until 1932 when Schlomka and Hinricks separated chest wall trauma induced injury into commotio cordis and contusion cordis [1, 2].

Commotio cordis, initially known as cardiac concussion or concussion of the heart, is derived from the Latin for disturbance of the heart. Commotio cordis has been defined as a condition of those victims who suffered from sudden death with a relatively minor (typically a thrown or batted baseball) chest wall injury and whose autopsies was shown no evidence of structural cardiac abnormalities or acute cardiac injury that could account for the sudden death [3].

That is to say, it occurs in structurally normal hearts without gross or microscopic injury to the myocardium, cardiac valves, or coronary arteries, as opposed to sudden cardiac death known to occur more frequently in contusion cordis.

Whereas contusion cordis is a term also derived from the Latin to describe direct pathologic injury to the heart and the thoracic cage, such as myocardial hemorrhage, coronary artery disruptions, rib fractures, et al., which occurred followed by high-energy chest wall impacts [4].

The Epidemiology of Commotio Cordis

Commotio cordis is a continuously rare event, and be apt to occur in male children, adolescents and youths.

At the first few years of the foundation of the commotio cordis of U.S. Minneapolis registry, only 70 victims of commotio cordis was documented [5]. With increasing public awareness of this phenomenon, the number of reported cases of commotio cordis has risen dramatically over the last few years. In the following ten years, the documented number of the victims of commotio cordis has increased to 154 cases [6].

Based on the records of the U.S. Consumer Product Safety Commission, the National Center for Catastrophic Sports Injury Research, and Little League Baseball, the demographic analysis of 25 victims of commotio cordis showed that the ages ranged from 3 to 19 years (with a mean of 11), and 72% were younger than 16 years. In addition, 96% of the victims were male, and only 1 subject was female, which showed predominantly striking difference [3]. Other demographic data also showed the similar tendency in age and sex [5, 6].

Commotio cordis has been reported in various sports, such as baseball, lacrosse, ice hockey, and softball, and as a consequence of fist fights, which may be the cause of being apt to occur in males [5, 7, 8].

The 182 fatal and non-fatal cases consecutively of commotio cordis entered into the U.S. Commotio Cordis Registry as of May 2006 were accessed, originated from the variety of sources, including news media, internet search engines, the LexisNexis database, the U.S.

Consumer Product Safety Commission, and submissions to the registry by medical examiners and other medical or sports related parties [9]. Of these 182 cases, 47% occurred during practice or competition in organized sports. These events occurred in baseball, lacrosse, hockey, and football.

Several years later, a systemic analysis about commotio cordis was performed in 2009. A registry of sudden deaths in young U.S. athletes (comprising 1866 systematically assembled cases) was a largely autopsy-based data set that encompasses events over a 27-year period from 1980 to 2006 in 38 organized sports performed at several competitive levels and provides insight into the number of such events that occur in trained athletes [10]. The incidence of commotio cordis in these athletes was 0.018/100 000 person-years. The low event rate should provide a measure of reassurance regarding sports participation but underscore the need for mandatory reporting of sudden deaths in young athletes, and it was also relevant to the question of whether a national screening program with noninvasive testing should be considered for U.S. athletes.

Due to its popularity in U.S., the number of victims during baseball is considerable. The U.S. Consumer Product Safety Commission report found 38 deaths from baseball blows to the chest between 1973 and 1995 [11]. Then focused on the commotio cordis, the initial record by the commotio cordis of U.S. Minneapolis registry, 128 victims from 1998 to September 2001 were documented. Of these cases, baseball accounted for 41% and softball 11%. For the past few years, commotio cordis is the second leading cause of death in youth athletics, occurring most frequently aged between 7 and 16 years in baseball but increasing also in lacrosse [12].

For the competitive lacrosse from 1980 to 2008, the U.S. National Registry of Sudden Death in Young Athletes was accessed. Of these 2015 athletes, ten athletes experienced precordial blows from the lacrosse ball or stick, which triggered commotio cordis, and four survived. During this period, high school and college lacrosse participation totaled 1578 872 person-years. The sudden death rate in lacrosse was 1.46 per 100 000 person-years, and greater significantly from the rates in some sports, including softball, track and field, and swimming. Nevertheless, commotio cordis events were disproportionately more common as a fraction of all of the deaths in lacrosse than in other sports. The commotio cordis sudden-death rate in lacrosse was 0.63 per 100 000 person-years, significantly greater than all of the other sports except hockey. Associated with the accelerated exposure of lacrosse has been a media focus on a number of recent deaths, particularly those attributed to commotio cordis [6].

Even most of the cases of commotio cordis were related to sports, fortunately, it is a rare event.

The Characteristics of Commotio Cordis

Based on the definition of commotio cordis, it is not difficult to see that the most prominent characteristic of commotio cordis is severe consequence followed by relatively minor chest wall blows.

Injury severity score (ISS) is an established medical score to assess trauma severity. It correlates with mortality, morbidity and hospitalization time after trauma. It is used to define the term major trauma, and it is based upon the Abbreviated Injury Scale (AIS). To calculate an ISS, take the highest AIS severity code in each of the three most severely injured ISS body regions, square each AIS code and add the three squared numbers for an ISS ($ISS=A^2+B^2+C^2$, where A, B, C are the AIS scores of the three most injured ISS body regions). The ISS scores ranges from 1 to 75. A major trauma or poly-trauma is defined as the ISS being greater than fifteen [13, 14]. But according to the narrow definition of commotio cordis, the ISS is only three. Even so, the mortality of commotio cordis is significantly higher than other victims with higher ISS.

However, the observed injuries were just present in the conduction system, which was able to cause the manifestations of heart block even seems minor. Link MS and colleges have found marked hemorrhage in the auriculo ventricular bundle and other bundle branches in 1 of 2 swine with transient heart block induced in their experimental model [15]. The injuries were not only found in the conduction system, but also in the myocardial fiber, not matter for the victims which were dead or alive. In another experimental model of commotio cordis, adult mongrel dogs were suffered from single impact at the velocity of 8.0 m/s effect on the precordial region at the sternum at the end of expiration with mechanical elastic-cord propelled impactor. The size of the impact interface of the shaft was 15.9 cm^2. The impact forces were simultaneously measured to range from 45.5 to 57.5 kg. Compared to the dogs in control group, macroscopically, no pericardial rupture, subepicardial hemorrhage as well as myocardial contusion at transverse sections were detected except for remarkable dilatation of subepicardial vessels. No injuries of the other viscera were identified at autopsy. Microscopic examination revealed no evident pathological changes other than slight or moderate waviness of myocardial fiber and the dilatation of small interstitial vessels in all the dogs impacted. Examined by the transmission electron microscopy, the ultra-structural imaging showed some myofibrils were relaxed with widened band, and some were over-contracted, thus showing contraction bands in all the dogs, and, the glycogen granules were abundant in cardiac cells in all the dogs, including the dogs in control group. Moreover, wavy myofibrils were present, and myofibrillar disrupture was occasionally present in only one dog [16]. In similar experimental research applied by rats, the histological examination of 13 days after blunt chest trauma with low-injury energy found the heart presented normal myocardium with mild congestion of included vessels [17]. In other words, it is demonstrated that some morphological changes might be present if detailed examinations were performed by more sophisticated or sensitive techniques in the cases of instantaneous death from commotio cordis.

The severe consequence of commotio cordis is instantaneous death due to ventricular fibrillation. But until now, the underlying mechanisms of cardiac arrest in commotio cordis have not been determined with certainty. Several theories have been advanced, involving ion channels, profound vasovagal reflex, and mechano-electrical coupling [18-21].

Ion channels are embedded in the cell membrane, which is directly bound to the myocardial cytoskeleton, which plays an integral role in maintaining cell shape and membrane stability. The profound electrophysiological consequences observed by Link MS were similar to those of myocardial ischemia, and then they hypothesized that the cellular mechanisms for arrhythmia in those two circumstances might be comparable. Based on the results of the experimental model of commotio cordis, selective K^+_{ATP} channel activation may be a pivotal mechanism in sudden death resulting from low-energy chest-wall trauma in young people during sporting activities [22].

K^+_{ATP} channels, which were discovered in the heart almost thirty years ago, serve as metabolic sensors that translate changes in cell metabolism into changes in electrical activity. In the heart, K^+_{ATP} channels are predominantly closed, but they may open in response to various forms of cardiac stress, including ischemia, physical exertion, stress hormones such as adrenaline, and mineralocorticoid-induced hypertension [23]. The opening K^+_{ATP} channels, which are associated with a reduction in the cellular ATP/ADP ration, lead to membrane hyperpolarization and shorten of the cardiac action potential, thereby reduce contractility, such as occurring in myocardial ischemia. In this way, K^+_{ATP} channels serve to reduce calcium influx and ATP consumption during metabolic stress. Because the membrane resistance is very high during the plateau of the cardiac action potential, opening of as few as 1% of the K^+_{ATP} channels in the cell can halve the cardiac action potential duration. Therefore, opening of K^+_{ATP} channels in response to stress and ischemia can be cardio-protective, yet gain-of-function mutations are associated with several pathologies, including congestive heart failure and Early Repolarization Syndrome, and so on [24, 25].

After application of glibenclamide, a selective inhibitor of the K^+_{ATP} channel, both on the QRS and before the T-wave peak in the swine model with chest impact, the incidence and severity levels of arrhythmia were significantly reduced. With QRS impacts, the maximal ST elevation was significantly less in those swine given glibenclamide, moreover, with T-wave impacts, the occurrences of ventricular fibrillation was significantly fewer in those swine given glibenclamide [22]. The detail of the reduction of arrhythmia is present in table 1. But it is a pity that this influential research about the mechanism of commotio cordis would not be applied in the emergency or much deeper research.

In other similar research, other stretch-sensitive ion channels, such as K^+_{Ach} calcium and other potassium, sodium and calcium channels have been described and could be involved in the incidence of commotio cordis [26-30]. Therefore, it is possible that these channels are activated by ventricular pressure increases and resultant myocardial stretch. A well-characterized stretch-activated channel (SAC) is the nonselective action channel, and it is present in mammalian and ovine species.

Table 1. Electrophysiological consequences of Low-energy chest impact in different conditions

Electrophysiological consequences	During the QRS segment		During the upslope of the T-wave	
	Without G	With G	Without G	With G
ST-segment elevation	0.35±0.20	0.16±0.10	0.07±0.04	0.11±0.07
Bundle branch block	90 %	100 %	25 %	15 %
Complete heart block	40 %	21 %	17 %	12 %
VF or PVT	0 %	0 %	33 %	4 %

* G represents for prior administration of gibenclamide; VF represents for ventricular fibrillation; PVT represents for polymorphic ventricular tachycardia.

This channel can be blocked by gadolinium, tarantula venom, or streptomycin. Blockade of this channel has been shown to reduce the frequency of stretch-induced arrhythmias. But the study showed no difference in the frequency of ventricular fibrillation in streptomycin-treated swine compared with the control swine, which was administered only sterile water. Moreover, no difference in the occurrence of polymorphic ventricular tachycardia was found.

However, the frequency and magnitude of ST segment elevation were reduced by blockade of the SAC with streptomycin. Such differences of the mechanism could help to explain why there are various kinds of cardiac arrhythmias occurred in different periods of the cardiac cycle [31].

There is an evidence to suggest that cytoskeleton might affect the cell membrane mechanical activation of ion channels [32]. With the same model, administration of colchicines, a well-known disruptor of the microtubular cytoskeleton, resulted in a significant increase in the incidence of ventricular fibrillation with chest wall impact [33]. Colchicine-pretreated swine had induced ventricular fibrillation at lower peak pressure rises compared with control animals. The present observation might be explained by a decrease in the rigidity of the cytoskeleton due to colchicines infusion resulting in an increase in the transmission of tensile forces as a result of mechanical stimulation. For the same left ventricular pressure achieved by chest impact there would be an expected increase in the opening for stretch-sensitive ion channels. The result influx of potassium ions across myocardial cell membranes alters repolarization and affects the predisposition to ventricular fibrillation. In conclusion, disruption of the cytoskeleton is likely to decrease cell membrane stiffness and increase deformation/stretch caused by left ventricular pressure rise. The mechanism of this increased activation may be increased membrane stretch secondary to loss of cytoskeleton scaffolding. In addition to cell membrane mechanism, intracellular signaling pathways may be also involved. G-protein activation can increase calcium signaling and predispose to arrhythmias via ryanodine receptor phosphorylation. In addition, a direct effect of colchicines on the opening of ion channels, or perhaps other proarrhythmic effects of the drug that remains to be determined.

Basic symptoms of commotio cordis range from brief palpitations to syncope and resuscitated sudden death. Presyncope and certainly syncope are more concerning, and resuscitated sudden death is of utmost worry. In the victims of commotio cordis, the presyncope always be transitory, and turns to certainly syncope promptly. Due to the fast development, syncope without prodromal symptoms and syncope at peak exercise are much more troubling than a gradual onset of syncope or syncope that is orthostatic or situational in nature. Syncope secondary to the injury during sports is more apt to occur in arrhythmic disorders and rarely occur in neurocardiogenic syncope. Frequent episodes of presyncope and lightheadness are less likely to be arrhythmic in origin than occasional episodes of syncope. Transient heart block may be the cause of episodes of syncope which result from a chest wall blow [15]. Vasovagal syncope is by far the most common cause of syncope and probably accounts for more than 50% of all episodes.

Because of the high sympathetic activity that is achieved while engaged in sporting activities, adrenergic tone has been cited as a possible mechanism by which ventricular fibrillation develops in commotio cordis victims. Beta-adrenergic blockade has been shown to decrease the occurrence of malignant ventricular arrhythmias and decrease mortality from ventricular tachycardia or fibrillation in humans and animals with recent myocardial infarction [34]. In consideration of vagotomy or medications and chest impacts which resulted in structural damage to the myocardium led to similar outcomes regardless of the presence or absence of vagal manipulation. In the classical experimental model of commotio cordis, the importance of the sympathetic and parasympathetic tone as important in the initiation of ventricular fibrillation and other cardiac arrhythmias was assessed. The result was not in accord with the previous hypothesis, moreover, it was the opposite. Indeed, the fact that the incidence of ventricular fibrillation, polymorphic ventricular tachycardia and the combined end-point ventricular fibrillation or polymorphic ventricular tachycardia were not affected by the administration of propranolol and atropine prior to chest wall blows suggests that sudden death due to commotio cordis involves alternative mechanisms. Vagotonic and sympathetic surges likely do not contribute to the syndrome of sudden death due to chest blows in youth. But the "trigger" that initiates a vasovagal reflex can be any of a number of different things. Pain is a particularly common cause of fainting. Sum up the clinical characteristics, it has been theorized that increased vagal tone, which occurs as a result of pain and fear after a chest wall blows, is the initiating event in commotio cordis.

Another theory about the mechanism of commotio cordis is mechano-electrical coupling. In animals, chest compressions can cause the phenomenon, which is the same as commotio cordis. Ventricular capture is defined as QRS complexes of similar morphology occurring intermittently but synchronized with the chest compressions artifact and impedance waveform. In the analysis of the patient who was suffered from cardiac arrest out-of-hospital, strong evidence that the mechanical force generated by chest compression in humans can cause ventricular capture was present, moreover, mechano-electrical coupling occurs in different settings with a wide range of externally applied mechanical forces, from precordial thumps to chest wall impact with projectile such as a baseball [35].

The Impact Factor of Incidence of Commotio Cordis

Studies about commotio cordis has changed from focus on epidemiology to experiment when a classical animal model was developed in 1998 [15]. However, Paul T considered swine was not suitable to be the animal model of commotio cordis due to its species-specific characteristics, because its prolongation of the QT interval might put swine at increased risk for ventricular fibrillation. According to their data, all ten young German Landrace pigs had ventricular fibrillation when radio-frequency current was delivered to the left ventricular myocardium. In these pigs, surface ECG showed a mean QT interval of 449±62.9 msec and a mean QT interval corrected for heart rate of 558.3±47.5 msec [36]. But Link MS and colleges firmly believed the experimental model of commotio cordis closely resembles the clinical profile of the catastrophic event. More specifically, the anatomy of pig is similar to that of humans and pigs were also chosen on the previous studies on chest-wall trauma.

The electrophysiologic consequences of impacts on the chest wall were critically dependent on the precise timing of the impact according to the cardiac cycle. The experiment showed that the ventricular fibrillation due to chest-wall impact only occurred during the 30-to-15-msec before the peak of the T wave, which was during cardiac repolarization. Therefore, the narrow vulnerable window is the crucial impact factor of the occurrence of commotio cordis, which might be the cause of that commotio cordis occurs as a rare event. Moreover, ventricular fibrillation is not preceded by intervening ventricular tachycardia, conduction abnormalities, or ischemic ST changes. Ventricular fibrillation produced by low-energy chest impact is not secondary to coronary spasm, myocardial ischemia, hemorrhage, heart block, or ventricular tachycardia, but rather is a primarily electrical phenomenon [22].

The cardiac rhythms initially identified in these victims were predominantly ventricular fibrillation, but complete heart block and idioventricular rhythm have also been reported [3, 19, 37]. Therefore, various arrhythmias might be present because of the chest blows occurred at different portions of the cardiac cycle. Of a total of ten blows during the 15-msec vulnerable window, nine produced ventricular fibrillation, which was consistently produced. Of course, in the present circumstance, ventricular fibrillation was no preceded by premature ventricular contractions, ischemia ST-segment changes, or heart block. Of the seven impacts during the T-wave, two brief bursts of polymorphic ventricular tachycardia occurred at thirteen and thirty-three msec before the T-wave peak, respectively. Of note, impacts during the QRS complex, four of ten were followed by transient and instantaneous complete heart block, which persisted for up to seven sinus beats, and others elicited immediate ST-segment elevation and left bundle-branch block, which was most likely due to epicardial coronary artery spasm, dissection, or thrombosis after excluding the presence of myocardial ischemia. Moreover, impacts during the ST-segment caused left bundle-branch block and associated or isolated ST-segment elevation. It was presumed to be that blunt impact on the chest wall of swine produced trauma to critical areas of the conduction system directly [15].

According to the epidemiological data, most of the reported cases of commotio cordis were related to baseball, and then the physical characteristics of the baseballs were tested to determine which mattered.

Initial study was about the hardness of the baseball grading by the reduced injury factor (RIF) [15]. A very soft safety ball (RIF 1) marked for use by children 5 to 7 years old, a medium soft ball (RIF 5) for use by children 8 to 10 years old, a least- soft ball (RIF 10) for use by children 11 an older, a standard regulation Little League baseball, and a wooden ball were included in the test. All the balls with the same mass were propelled at the same velocity with 48 km/h. The results showed that significant differences in the induction of ventricular fibrillation between the softest safety ball and the regulation ball and between the wooden object and each of the baseballs. But no significant differences were evident between the regulation baseball and the medium soft and the least soft safety baseballs.

Apart of the foregoing impact factors, the impact energy of the baseball effecting on the chest to generate ventricular fibrillation is also very crucial [38]. Applied by the classical experimental model, they found that the ventricular fibrillation could not be induced with 20 impacts mph, the incidence of ventricular fibrillation increased incrementally from 7% with 25 mph impact, to 68% with 40 mph impacts, and then diminished at more than 50 mph. Then, an apparent paradox generated, which was about the cause of higher-velocity impacts be less apt to induce commotio cordis related ventricular fibrillation. In the study, papillary muscle tears and left ventricular wall rupture first occurred at 50 mph and increased to 77% with 70 mph blows, indicating that at such high velocities it often created contusion cordis, but not commotio cordis.

Moreover, the peak left ventricular pressure generated by the impact effect on the chest was associated with the incidence of ventricular fibrillation in a similar Gaussian relationship. Compared with ventricular fibrillation, the incidence of transient complete heart block, bundle branch block, and ST segment elevation increased incrementally relative to the velocities of impact and best fit a linear curve. That is to say, the energy of impact is an important factor in the generation of ventricular fibrillation with chest-wall impacts. Impacts at 40 mph were more apt to induce ventricular fibrillation than impacts with greater or lesser velocities, suggesting that the predilection for commotio cordis is related in a complex manner to the precise velocity of chest-wall impact. Then, with the relatively specific quality and velocity, it is not hard to evaluate the predilection of energy to trigger commotio cordis.

Another significant impact factor of commotio cordis is the location of the impact. Summary of the victims suggested the lethal impacts effect on the precordium, but the precise location of impact relative to the risk of sudden death had not clarified until the research by Link MS in 2001 [39]. Applying by the previous experimental model, the results suggested that ventricular fibrillation was only triggered by impacts directly over the cardiac silhouette, such as the center of the left ventricle, the apex of the left ventricle, and the base of the left ventricle, furthermore, impact directly over the center of the heart showed more frequently apt to be fatal than were those at the periphery of the heart. Other cardiac arrhythmias, such as ST segment elevation, nonsustained polymorphic ventricular tachycardia, transient heart block, or bundle branch block, were also occurred only with impacts directly over the cardiac silhouette in not causing ventricular fibrillation situation. Compared with noncardiac sites, including the left lateral, left posterior, right posterior, and right lateral chest wall, peak left ventricle pressure became markedly elevated as an immediate consequence of impact directly over the cardiac silhouette. Based on the univariate logistic regression model, temporal change in left ventricular pressure (DP/DT) occurred as a result of impact to be highly predictive of the initiation of ventricular fibrillation; moreover, DP/DT was highest in the impact at the center of the left ventricle, and decreased relative to the distance of the impact from the center of the left ventricle, in other words, the magnitude and rate of the rise were associated with the risk for ventricular fibrillation. And that the left ventricular wall motion abnormalities resulted only from impacts directly over the cardiac silhouette. Regional mechanical and electrophysiological changes accompany most ventricular arrhythmias and, it has been suggested, by mechano-electric feedback. Because Waldman and colleges had found that three principal strain components at a given region of the left ventricle did not always align themselves with the local fiber direction, the electrical and mechanical behavior of the thin-walled right ventricle was then systematically studied based on the lambs model, due to right ventricle is an irregular crescent-shaped chamber and its inflow and outflow tracts differ with respect to origin, morphology, innervations, and function [40, 41]. Increased mechanical loading of the heart is often related to arrhythmias, the so-called "stretch-induced arrhythimas", which is one relatively undisputed mechanical cause of arrhythmia during commotio cordis. For the mechanically induced arrhythmias, dispersion in repolarization time could promote regional current flow and reentry mechanisms. Early afterdepolarization increased the amplitude and duration after the increase of right ventricle pressure and regional segment length during pulmonary artery occlusion, and the increase of the amplitude of early afterdepolarization was linearly and positively related to the increase of the corresponding regional segment length. These early afterdepolarizations were strongly related to right ventricle premature beats. Pulmonary artery occlusions would be apt to give rise to a variety of right ventricular arrhythmias, such as PVBs, bigemini, salvos, and ventricular tachycardia, but none progressed to be ventricular fibrillation. Early afterdepolarization may precipitate arrhythmia in the following two ways. One is that if the magnitude of early afterdepolarization exceeds a threshold excitation, it may directly induce premature beats causing a type of trigger activity. Another is that if one area has a marked early afterdepolarization and a prolonged monophasic action potential duration at 90% repolarization ($MAPD_{90}$) and therefore a refractory period while another area has a reduce $MAPD_{90}$ and a refractory period, which could increase electrophysiological dispersion that favors the development of reentry and/or predisposes activation of abnormal current flow between the two areas. However, whether the early afterdepolarization has effected on the ventricular fibrillation during commotio cordis, it need to be proved in the future.

According to the Product Summary Report, sixty-eight of eighty-eight fatalities were related to baseball impacts [42]. According to another recent report, eighteen of twenty-five individuals were documented in baseball or softball. In an effort to reduce injuries in different sports, protective equipment has been perfected and mandated for some sporting events. Certain sports, such as football, require protective gear such as chest, leg, and arm pads as well as an approved helmet. Other sports with less person-to-person contact only require a minor amount of equipment. Such as baseball and softball, only a batting helmet as protective equipment was required for players while batting. In particular, catchers are required to wear more extensive protection because of their close proximity to the pitched balls. For different sexes, females are required to equipment pelvic protector to provide groin protection against impact, and, males are required to wear athletic cup to provide groin and testicle protection against impact. In consideration of the impact region of commotio cordis, batting vests have gained more attention for injury protection during baseball sports. Even the vests became more developed, the fact that 28% of the victims were wearing different type of chest protector and still died from commotio cordis raises a question as to the protective effectiveness of current vests in baseball [3].

To correlate impact energy to a risk of injury, researchers have explored various injury criteria. The risk of blunt trauma to the thorax has been assessed by using an empirically based injury criterion called the viscous criterion (VC), which accurately predicts the risk of vital organ and soft tissue injury when other criteria fail. The criterion has used extensively for motor vehicle occupants to predict the severity of injury. The viscous criterion is calculated based on the amount of thoracic compression and the velocity at which this compression occurs. The amount of thoracic compression was defined as the displacement of the chest in relationship to the spine normalized by the initial thickness of the thorax. A tolerable level of chest compression at a low velocity can prove to be fatal at higher velocities of deformation. Viscous criterion has been validated as a useful tool in determining injury severity related to blunt ballistic impacts to the thorax and predicting life-threatening cardiac arrhythmias. The rate-sensitive tolerable compression leads to the introduction of the VC, VCmax, which accounts for the importance of both parameters during commotio cordis, including the velocity of deformation and compression [43]. Therefore, the introduction of viscous criterion to evaluate the definite energy of the chest blow may be beneficial to explore the impact factor of commotio cordis and to test the effect of chest protectors.

A novel test methodology has been developed by Wayne State University for the purpose of evaluating the effectiveness of chest protectors in reducing the risk of commotio cordis. A device was developed utilizing the ribs from the BioSID (First Technology Safety Systems, Farmington, MI) crash dummy utilized for side impact tests in the automotive research community. The device is recently validated for blunt ballistic impacts using masses and impact velocities similar to those of the baseball impacts. Therefore, this system is ideal for the blunt chest impacts, since the rib structure is continuous at the impact side, thus providing an adequately uniform loading surface for the concentrated impacts of a baseball or other softballs to the chest [44, 45]. Briefly speaking, the main part of the device is three-rib chest structure (3-RCS). 3-RCS involves three thoracic ribs mounted to a spine box opposite the impact point. Dampening material on the inside of the rib provides for viscous bending resistance and dissipates energy. Nylon supports are mounted to the sides of the spine box to prohibit upward and downward motion of the ribs. A urethane bib tied the three ribs together on the impact side. A position transducer was mounted to the interior of the ribs in the anteroposterior position to measure the amount of chest deflection of the middle rib. The transducer was connected directly behind the urethane bib in the sternal region. The base of the transducer was mounted within the spine box. This arrangement allowed measurement of chest displacement. The linearity of the position transducer was verified statistically over a range of 50 mm and dynamically for velocities up to 10 m/s by manufacturer's specifications. Differentiation of the rib displacement was used to verify that the velocity of deformation did not exceed this level during testing. Calibration tests with the three-rib system demonstrated an average 6.8% coefficient of variation in viscous criterion and 3.4% in chest deflection for 11 tests with 2.3% coefficient of variation in impact speeds [46]. The chest structure was placed on a free-moving sled to allow unrestricted horizontal movement with each impact, simulating whole-body motion in an impact. Spine mass reflects torso inertia effects. A pressurized air cannon was used to propel a standard baseball placed approximately 50 cm from the 3-RCS. The sled was repositioned to the same starting point after each impact, and the amount of displacement of the entire system was recorded to reflect momentum exchange to the 3-RCS [47].

Historically, the purpose of chest protectors was to reduce the sting of baseball impacts to the chest as well as to lessen the potential for various levels of injuries. Vests might not have been optimized to the dual need for pain and fatal arrhythmia prevention. Tested by the mechanical model, most commercially available vests had lower viscous criterion at different grades, such as All Star vest, ASP vest, and the West vest. However, the IPASC vest presented bad protective effect, involving a 34.2% increase in viscous criterion. Due to the analysis of mechanical characteristic of vest, there are several ways in which a vest can reduce the energy transfer to the chest. One is to spread the impact load over a greater area of the chest, which could lower the local pressure of impact and reduces chest deflection. Another is to absorb a portion of the kinetic energy of impact. Materials that have the greatest energy absorption versus elastically storing the deformation energy can effectively reduce the energy transfer to the chest. The third is from the mass of the vest. During impact, the local mass of the vest must be accelerated until the ball reaches common velocity with the interface. Moreover, it is likely that a combination of effects is occurring in baseball, such as when the impact coincides with the vulnerable phase of the T-wave and when the protective effects of the vest do not sufficiently lower energy transfer to the chest. But inevitably there are amount of assumptions and additional factors that influence the estimation of field benefits from sports equipment tested in the laboratory. According to the previous results, even the protective vest will not prevent all cases of commotio cordis, the methodology and analysis procedure of the test offer a means to further improve the performance of chest protectors used in baseball, moreover, improvements in materials and design of chest wall barriers are necessary to reduce the occurrence of these tragic events and make the athletic field safer for youths.

For the same purpose, the frequency of ventricular fibrillation that resulted from chest wall blows with baseballs and lacrosse balls was analyzed. Applied by the classical experimental model, the unenthusiastic result was present. The commercially available baseball and lacrosse chest wall protectors were ineffective in protecting against ventricular fibrillation that was triggered by chest blows and, by inference, sudden cardiac death [48].

Fortunately, the baseball chest protectors were not good for nothing. 42.9% of chest protectors could lower mean left ventricular pressures, and 28.6% of chest protectors were associated with significantly less ST segment elevation. However, no significant reduction in the occurrence of bundle branch block was attributable to any of the baseball chest protectors. For the lacrosse chest protectors, 42.9% could lower mean maximum left ventricular pressure, 28.6% were associated with significantly less ST segment elevation, moreover, 85.7% had significantly lower frequency of bundle branch block. Of note, a trend toward protection from ventricular fibrillation as induced by chest impacts with lacrosse balls was present in only one particular chest barrier, which was composed of a layer that contained sleeves of expanded polypropylene beads, a unique material composition that was not found in other available products. Moreover, none of the impact to the right or left posterior or lateral chest walls was related to the alteration in left ventricular function. Based on the experimental data, chest wall protection need not extend to the right chest wall, the back or to other areas of the chest distant from the heart.

As mentioned above, experimental impacts to anesthetized swine have been developed because there were cases of ventricular fibrillation without serious injury to the heart, lungs, and internal organs. These cases could reflect the predominant characteristic for commotio cordis. Ventricular fibrillation is defined as a rapid polymorphic ventricular arrhythmia that required defibrillation. By definition, there is a significant statistical correlation between ventricular fibrillation and viscous criterion from those tests, and a logical injury risk function could be determined.

Not only could the chest suffering from blunt impact induce commotio cordis, but also could the back. Therefore, to strengthen of chest protectors to a point could reduce the risk of commotio cordis.

The Diagnosis of Commotio Cordis

As mentioned above, commotio cordis is a rare event, and it aggregates to be dead within several minutes, therefore, there is less information to aid the diagnosis.

More and more cases of commotio cordis were reported, then Jackimczyk K concluded commotio cordis might occur under the following circumstances: an abrupt deceleration injury causing the heart to impact against the sternum and a crash injury of the chest, which either compressed the heart between the sternum and thoracic vertebrae or caused damage to the heart by increasing intrathoracic pressure transmitted against a closed glottis [49].

But due to its complexity, there is no generally accepted diagnostic criterion for commotio cordis until 2002. Based on the conclusion of most of cases of commotio cordis, each case fulfilled these inclusion criteria: (1) a witnessed occurrence of a blunt, non-penetrating chest blow immediately preceding cardiovascular collapse; (2) documentation of the circumstances of the event; and (3) the absence of structural damage to the sternum, ribs, and heart itself or underlying cardiovascular abnormalities at autopsy [3, 50].

Even it is so difficult, many different approaches have been used in the diagnosis of potentially serious cardiac blunt trauma, including chest radiography, ECG, echocardiography, computed tomographic scanning, radionuclide imaging, and enzyme analysis, such as CK-MB and cardiac troponins T and I. But the optimal methods of evaluation remain unclear.

The electrocardiogram (ECG) is the efficient technology to monitor the arrhythmias in clinical practice. But the ECG of commotio cordis is nonspecific, repolarization abnormalities are always common, and then tend to change rapidly. Arrhythmias are frequently the mechanism of death following commotio cordis. According to the data of an experimental animal studies, arrhythmias occurred in up to 50% of the cases [51]. Disturbances in cardiac rhythm include frequent atrial arrhythmias and ventricular extrasystoles and bundle branch blocks or atrioventricular conduction disturbances that may result in complete heart block.

Link MS has reported the detailed medical data of a survivor. The initial ECG showed marked ST elevation in the anterior leads. ST abnormalities persisted into the fourth day with gradual decline to baseline. Q waves never developed and the QTc interval was always within normal limits [52]. No matter the real cases, or the experimental model, the ECG were widely different, ranging from minor ST elevation to fatal ventricular fibrillation, even worse, no specific arrhythmia was exclusive for commotio cordis.

Other technology and biochemistry markers are still in the research, but not the practice. Then appropriate method chosen might be according to the definition of commotio cordis. The pathological findings of the commotio cordis identified by the forensic pathologists may be the most crucial but complex part. According to the animal model, no animal after impact had rib fractures, hemothorax, hemopericardium, or evidence of myocardial contusion, which were distinctly excluded in the diagnosis of commotio cordis. However, minor injuries were always confused in the diagnosis. The moderate degree of hemorrhage in the anterior left ventricle also could be present even in the swine from control group. For the conduction system, marked hemorrhage of the atrioventricular bundle and bundle branches could be present in swine with heart block, and mild hemorrhage was present in each of the swine with ventricular fibrillation [15].

In some reported cases of commotio cordis, injuries or underlying cardiovascular diseases with different degrees were also present. Marshall DT reported a case of commotio cordis associated with a single vehicle roll-over accident. The victim had enlarged and dilated heart, weighting 491 g, and a focal area of atherosclerosis was found in the left anterior descending coronary artery causing 50% stenosis [53]. Miyazaki T also reported a case of commotio cordis associated with a traffic accident. A transverse 4 cm long tear of the ascending aorta 1 cm distal from the origin of the aorta with adventitial hematoma was presents [54]. Apart from the occurrence of commotio cordis, only the atherosclerosis with 50% stenosis or mild tears of the aorta could be the causes of death.

Based on the circumstantial evidence, eyewitness accounts, the defendant's statements, temporal sequence of events, the lack of an impact injury on the front or lack of the chest, and the negative autopsy findings and post-mortem drug screen, the cause of death was identified as commotio cordis.

Without the result of gene screening, some other diseases are also similar to commotio cordis. Also uncommonly occurred in the athlete, Brugada Syndrome also presents fatal ventricular arrhythmias and sudden cardiac death in normal structural heart. Although few of the victims were electrocardiographically monitored at the time of death, most of the sudden deaths were thought to be due to ventricular arrhythmias, especially ventricular fibrillation.

In idiopathic ventricular fibrillation, a significant subset of individuals suffering from the Brugada Syndrome, which is secondary to an abnormality of the SCN5A channel.

Consideration should be given to a flecainide challenge to accentuate the ECG changes found in the Brugada Syndrome. Brugada syndrome is a tutosomal dominant, cardiac sodium channelopathy, which clinically presents with syncope or less commonly as ventricular fibrillation leading to sudden cardiac death. An ECG pattern of J-point and ST segment elevation in the right precordial leads is typically seen. Mixed phenotypic expressions of the disease, ranging from distince repolarisation to subclinical cardiac conduction defects, also occur. Increased vagal tone induced by chronic athletic conditioning may enhance the propensity to die at rest, and hyperthermia during exercise may potentially trigger arrhythmias during strenuous activity [55].

Due to the common characteristics, more should be performed to do the differential diagnosis of Brugada Syndrome and commotio cordis. The key elements of the diagnosis include the severity of the symptoms, the presence or absence of structural heart disease, and the family medical history.

Moreover, the differential diagnosis of anomalous coronary arteries and commotio cordis is another difficulty and might require cardiac catheterization. Anomalous coronary arteries can be suggested by syncope at peak exercise, or ischemia on exercise testing. Most of the victims involving in anomalous coronary arteries present with exertion.

The Treatment of Commotio Cordis

Commotio cordis generally is fatal, with survival in only 15 % of cases [56]. When survival presents, usually it is related to the rapid initiation of resuscitation and occasionally a precordial thump.

During cardiopulmonary resuscitation, ventricular fibrillation frequently recurs and is thought to be a marker of a poor outcome. The current American Heart Association Guidelines for cardiopulmonary resuscitation recommend a 1-shock protocol with immediate resumption of chest compression, minimizing the "no-flow" time, which is known to adversely affect the outcomes. Unfortunately, it is not possible to obtain continuous intra-cardiac electrical recordings during out-of-hospital CPR. The incidence of ventricular capture caused by chest compressions might have been underestimated if chest compression and ventricular capture occurred in a 1:1 ratio, and a correlation between ventricular capture and survival could not be made [57]. However, CPR was treated as the effective approach to increase the proportion of survivors.

Timely resuscitative efforts have been shown to improve survival up to 58% within the last six years, whereas resuscitative delays more than three minutes are related to survival of only 3%. For the survival rate of the victims of commotio cordis, it is getting higher owing to more rapid response times and access to defibrillation, as well as greater public awareness according to a recent study [58]. In previous cases, resuscitative efforts were often significantly delayed, due to lack of awareness by the bystanders that the chest blows were sufficient to trigger cardiac arrest. In contrast, 3 of 25 incidents forming the survivors report involved particularly rapid institution of resuscitative measures by trained bystanders (within 15 seconds, 1minute, and 3 minute), and it is likely that this prompt response was a major determinant of survival [59]. In summary, recognizing the present rare syndrome is the predominant. Second, more rapid CRP implementation, more survival possibility is gained. Third, the CRP would be better implemented by trainee, such as physician, or lifeguard, et al.

An automated external defibrillator (AED) is a portable device that checks the heart rhythm. If needed, it can send an electric shock to the heart to try to restore a normal rhythm. In a retrospective study, Cecchin and colleges analyzed ECGs from children aged 12 years or younger and found a sensitivity of 96% for ventricular fibrillation and a specificity of 100% for nonshokcbale rhythms [60]. Moreover, AEDs could be used to treat sudden cardiac arrest, which is common in commotio cordis. However, according to the current guideline of American Heart Association, the AED presently is recommended for use only in individuals who is eight years old or older. But about 25% of victims who suffered from commotio cordis are younger than eight years. Therefore, an evident paradox related to the use of AED as a therapy for ventricular fibrillation in commotio cordis is present. Applied by the classical experimental model, the sensitivity, specificity, and survival rate of AED therapy of commotio cordis were assessed. In the research, successful defibrillation was defined as an AED shock that terminated ventricular fibrillation. The sensitivity for initial detection in each of the instances the AED appropriately diagnosed ventricular fibrillation was 100%, and the specificity of that was also 100%. Thus, the AED did not call for defibrillation in any of the non-ventricular fibrillation ECG segments. Refer to the defibrillation, the successful rate of AED therapy of ventricular fibrillation was 100%, including first shock defibrillation efficacy occurred in 94% ventricular fibrillation inductions, two shocks occurred in 4%, and three shocks occurred in 2%. The foregoing survival rate of AED therapy of commotio cordis was 100%, but defibrillation was achieved at the premise of fibrillation only lasted less than 1 minute. For those at 2 minutes, the survival rate decreased to 92%, and for those at 4 minutes, and the survival rate decreased to 46% and for those at 6 minutes of ventricular fibrillation, the survival rate was further to 25%. The result suggests that earlier defibrillation would improve survival rates in commotio cordis, and more universal AED use would represent a key element in achieving the consequence [61].

The high sensitivity and specificity suggested that there was a very low risk of an inappropriate shock with the optimal dose of defibrillation energy and that the AED correctly identified shockable rhythms, making the algorithm both safe and effective for children. Fortunately, AED using pads that decrease shock energy to 50 J has been approved by the U.S. Food and Drug Administration for pediatric use, and then with the device, it would allow defibrillation energies closer to the recommended 2 J/kg for most children [62].

Another issue limiting more universal AED use in young children might be the relatively low incidence of ventricular fibrillation reported in association with sudden death in the pediatric age group. However, the commotio cordis is apparently rare involving in reports of cardiac arrest in adult victims.

Link MS and colleges thought the commotio cordis not only might be secondary to ventricular fibrillation, but also might be associated with coronary vasospasm or segmental changes in myocardial contractility through observation of the clinical, angiographic, and hemodynamic date of a rare survivor [52]. This founding might make the rapid rescue measurements more crucial to decrease in fatal events.

Not only is low the survival rate, unfortunately, but also various complications about different victims of commotio cordis were reported. The prognosis for commotio cordis is good if the patient survives the first 24 hours. Generally speaking, if rhythm disturbances do not occur by the second day, this complication no longer needs to be considered. But if rhythm disturbances occur, they can last for weeks. Most of them suffered from various complications with different grades even in several years later.

Among the survivals, only a few were fortunate, who remained stable without apparent psychological or neurologic deficit or cardiac symptoms, and there was no evidence of structural cardiovascular disease. Some survivors were more or less had neurologic deficit due to anoxic encephalopathy, manifested by a moderate physical and neurologic impairment, requiring assistance with quantitative concepts, or manifested by a mild spastic paralysis and a moderate memory loss, or worse to be mild cognitive and visual-spatial impairment. Compared with their long-term consequences, their sub-chronic complications were even worse. They remained comatose and dependent on mechanical ventilation or could not regain full consciousness for several or dozens of days [52, 59].

The Preventive Strategies of Commotio Cordis

As there is no single approach for the complex problem, the search for the optimal strategy to decrease the occurrence of sudden cardiac death due to commotio cordis in young athletes is only raising the curtain.

Due to the high occurrence rate of commotio cordis during competitive or recreational baseball, safety of the balls and effectiveness of the protective vest were tested to improve. Of 182 cases of commotio cordis, 18% were related to fatal chest blows despite the presence of potentially protective equipment [9]. Even the athletes wore standard, commercially available chest barriers made of polymer foam covered by fabric or hard shells, generally perceived as protective from arrhythmic consequences of the blows. Scenarios included the failure of the padding to cover the precordium region so that blows circumvented the protective barrier or projectiles that struck the chest barrier directly.

Based on the foregoing reported data, the hardness, sizes, shapes of the baseball should be paid more attention during the design and producing to reduce the occurrence of commotio cordis. The use of safety baseballs has been recommended by the Consumer Product Safety Commission as a way to decrease the occurrence of injuries in youth baseball. Whereas, dispute are still continued about whether softer baseballs are beneficial to lower risk of commotio cordis. Janda DH and colleges considered that the risk of commotio cordis might be increased by the softer baseball as compared with the regular baseball [63]. But Link MS and colleges have opposite opinion, which was that softest baseball was associated with lowest risk of producing ventricular fibrillation [15]. In another word, the medium soft and least soft baseballs might be suitable for play in the older age groups, but whether these baseballs would lower the risk of commotio cordis in actual play need determined in the further research.

Moreover, the use and improvement of protective vest might be another focus to avoid the catastrophe as far as possible, even though the universal use of commercial chest protectors has not been advised due to insufficient evidence regarding their benefit. However, when commotio cordis occurs despite the use of a chest protector, the event is especially troubling, given the false sense of security that is conveyed unintentionally by wearing the commercially available barrier. And then, novel materials and design that are effective in dissipating impact energy in time and space differently from barriers that are designed to protect against tissue injury may be necessary to achieve this goal. Based on this requirement, a novel design of protective equipment to minimize trauma-related deaths has been developed [64].

Prevention of commotio cordis can be aided by the general increase in public awareness that an impact to the chest can result in sudden death, and then second preventive strategies should also be paid attention, such as timely CPR by the trained persons if permitted, and timely AED. The on-site AED programming at sport venues has been implemented as secondary prevention strategy in the USA, and then expert advised that implementation for similar programmer in Europe, fully realizing that spectators as well as athletes may benefit [65]. Public and policy efforts to provide AEDs at sports events may improve the chance for meaningful survival after occurrence of commotio cordis. For victims who survive commotio cordis, neither invasive testing nor ICD implantation are generally indicated, although noninvasive testing with 12-lead ECG, Holter monitoring, and echocardiography is advised [66]. The foregoing medical strategies, strictly speaking, were not specific for commotio cordis, which are just for restore the sinus arrhythmia.

In fact, there are still no definite, specific and effective preventive strategies to prevent the occurrence of commotio cordis. The most important is extensive known about commotio cordis, especially in the sports community and medical community. Therefore, more athletes would try their best to reduce the occurrence of commotio cordis, and more trained bystanders or first-aid personals would do all they can to increase the survival rate of commotio cordis.

Acknowledgments

This chapter is partially supported by the grants from NSFC (81102302, 81202529, 31171096).

References

[1] Glinz W. Injuries to the heart by blunt trauma. In: Glinz W. Chest trauma: diagnosis and management. *Berlin: Springer-Verlag*. 1981; 191-203.

[2] Schlomka G, Hinrichs A. Experimentelle Untersuchungen über den Einfluss stumpfer Brustkorbverletzungen auf das Elektrokardiogram. *Z. Gesamte. Exp. Med.* 1932; 81:43-61.

[3] Maron BJ, Poliac LC, Kaplan JA, et al. Blunt impact to the chest leading to sudden death from cardiac arrest during sports activities. *N. Engl. J. Med.* 1995; 333:337-42.

[4] Kalin JA, Madias C, Link MS. Prevention of sudden cardiac death: commotio cordis. In: Douglas JC. Preventing sudden death in sport and physical activity. Burlington: *Jones & Bartlett Learning*. 2012; 43.

[5] Maron BJ, Link MS, Wang PJ, et al. Clinical profile of commotio cordis: an underappreciated cause of sudden death in the young during sports and other adtivities. *J. Cardiovasc. Eletrophysiol.* 1999; 10:114-120.

[6] Maron BJ, Doerer JJ, Haas TS, et al. Commotio cordis and the epidemiology of sudden death in competitive lacrosse. *Pediatrics*. 2009; 124:966-71.
[7] Zheng N, Liang M, Liu Y, et al. Commotio cordis—a report of two similar cases. *J. Forensic. Sci*. 2013; 58:245-7.
[8] Zheng N, Liang M, Liu Y, et al. Imprudent blow, catastrophic consequence: a case of commotio cordis associated with violence. *Med. Sci. Law*. 2012; 52:119-21.
[9] Doerer JJ, Haas TS, Estes NAM 3rd. Evaluation of chest barriers for protection against sudden death due to commotio cordis. *Am. J. Cardiol*. 2007; 99:857-9.
[10] Maron BJ, Doerer JJ, Haas TS, et al. Sudden death in young competitive athletes analysis of 1866 deaths in the United States, 1980-2006. *Circulation*. 2009; 119:1085-92.
[11] Adler P, Monticone RCJ. Injuries and deaths related to baseball. In: Kyle SB. Youth Baseball Protective Equipment Project: Final Report. Washington DC: *U.S. Consumer Product Safety Commission*. 1996; 1-43.
[12] Maron BJ. Sudden death in young athletes. *N. Engl. J. Med*. 2003; 349:1064-75.
[13] Keel M, Trentz O. Pathophysiology of polytrauma. *Injury*. 2005; 36:691-709.
[14] Copes WS, Champion HR, Sacco WJ, et al. The injury severity score revisted. *J. Trauma*. 1988; 28:69-77.
[15] Link MS, Wang PJ, Pandian NG, et al. An experimental model of sudden death due to low-energy chest-wall impact (commotio cordis). *N. Eng. J. Med*. 1998; 338:1805-11.
[16] Guan DW, Ohshima T, Jia JT, et al. Morphological findings of 'cardiac concussion' due to experimental blunt impact to the precordial region. *Forensic. Sci. Int*. 1999; 100:211-20.
[17] Wang ND, Stevens MH, Doty DB, et al. Blunt chest trauma: an experimental model for heart and lung contusion. *J. Trauma*, 2003; 54744-8.
[18] Viano DC, Andrzejak DV, King AI. Fatal chest injury by baseball impact in children. *Clin. J. Sport Med*. 1992; 2:161-5.
[19] Kaplan JA, Karofsky PS, Volturo GA. Commotio cordis in two amateur ice hockey players despite the use of commercial chest protectors: case reports. *J. Trauma*. 1993; 34:151-3.
[20] Viano DC, Andraejak DV, Polley TZ, et al. Mechanism of fatal chest injury by baseball impact development of an experimental model. *Clin. J. Sport Med*. 1992; 2:166-71.
[21] Wang JN, Tsai YC, Chen SL, et al. Dangerous impact-commotio cordis. *Cardiology*. 2000; 93:124-6.
[22] Link MS, Wang PJ, VanderBrink BA, et al. Selective activation of the K^+_{ATP} channel is a mechanism by which sudden death is produced by low-energy chest-wall impact (commotio cordis). *Circulation*. 1999; 100:413-8.
[23] Kane GC, Liu XK, Yamada S, et al. Cardiac KATP channels in health and disease. *J. Mol. Cell Cardiol*. 2005; 38:937-43.
[24] Faivre JF, Findlay I. Action potential duration and activation of ATP-sensitive potassium current in isolated guinea-pig ventricular myocytes. *Biochim. Biophys. Acta*. 1990; 1029:167-72.
[25] Zhang HX, Silva JR, Nichols CG. Cardiac K_{ATP} channels in health and disease. In: Gussak I, Antzelevitch C. Electrical diseases of the heart, 2nd edition. London: *Springer*. 2013; 259-79.

[26] Hu H, Sachs F. Stretch-activated ion channels in the heart. *J. Mol. Cell Cardiol.* 1997; 29:1511-23.

[27] Pleumsamran A, Kim D. Membrane stretch augments the cardiac muscarinic K+ channel activity. *J. Membrane Biol.* 1995; 148:287-97.

[28] Matsuda N, Hagiwara N, Shoda M, et al. Enhancement of the L-type Ca^{2+} current by mechanical stimulation in single rabbit cardiac myocytes. *Circ. Res.* 1996; 78:650-9.

[29] Gannier F, White E, Lacampagne A, et al. Streptomycin reverses a large stretch induced increase in Ca^{2+} in isolated guinea pig ventricular myocytes. *Carciovasc. Res.* 1994; 28:1193-8.

[30] Ruknudin A, Sachs F, Bustamante JO. Stretch-activated ion channels in tissue-cultured chick heart. *Am. J. Physiol.* 1993; 264:H960-72.

[31] Garan AR, Maron BJ, Wang PJ, et al. Role of streptomycin-sensitive stretch-activated channel in chest wall impact induced sudden death (commotio cordis). *J. Cardiovasc. Electrophysiol.* 2005; 16:433-8.

[32] Janmey PA. The cytoskeleton and cell signaling: component localization and mechanical coupling. *Physiol. Rev.* 1998; 78:763-81.

[33] Madias C, Maron BJ, Supron S, et al. Cell membrane: stretch and chest blow-induced ventricular fibrillation: commotio cordis. *J. Cardiovasc. Electrophysio.* 2008; 19: 1304-9.

[34] Hjalmarson A, Olsson G. Myocardial infarction. Effects of beta-blockade. *Circulation.* 1991; 84:V1101-7.

[35] Cayla G, Macia JC, Pasquie JL. Images in cardiovascular medicine: precordial thump in the catheterization laboratory experimental evidence for commotio cordis. *Circulation.* 2007; 115:e332.

[36] Paul T, Bökenkamp R, Mahnert B, et al. Coronary artery involvement early and late after radiofrequency current application in young pigs. *Am. Heart J.* 1997; 133:436-40.

[37] Green ED, Simson LR Jr, Kellerman HH, et al. Cardiac concussion following softball blow to the chest. *Ann. Emerg. Med.* 1980; 9:155-7.

[38] Link MS, Maron BJ, Wang PJ, et al. Upper and lower energy limits of vulnerability to sudden death with chest wall impact (commotio cordis). *J. Am. Coll. Cardiol.* 2003; 41:99-104.

[39] Link MS, Maron BJ, VanderBrink BA, et al. Impact directly over the cardiac silhouette is necessary to produce ventricular fibrillation in an experimental model of commotio cordis. *J. Am. Coll. Cardiol.* 2001; 37:649-54.

[40] Waldman LK, Fung YC, Covell JW. Transmural myocardial deformation in the left ventricle. *Circ. Res.* 1985; 57:152-63.

[41] Chen RL, Penny DJ, Greve G, et al. Stretch-induced regional mechanoelectric dispersion and arrhythmia in the right ventricle of anesthetized lambs. *Am. J. Physiol. Heart Circ. Physiol.* 2004; 286:H1008-14.

[42] NEISS. Product Summary Report. Washington. DC: *Consumer Product Safety Commission.* 1996;1983.

[43] Viano DC, Lau IV. A viscous tolerance criterion for soft tissue injury assessment. *J. Biomech.* 1988; 21:387-99.

[44] Bir C, Viano D, King A. Development of biomechanical response corridors of the thorax to blunt ballistic impacts. *J. Biomech.* 2004; 37:73-9.

[45] Bir CA. The evaluation of blunt ballistic impacts of the thorax. Detroit: *Wayne State University*. Doctoral dissertation. 2000; 54-62.

[46] Janda DH, Bir CA, Viano DC, et al. Blunt chest impacts: assessing the relative risk of fatal cardiac injury from various baseballs. *J. Trauma*. 1998; 44:298-303.

[47] Viano DC, Bir CA, Cheney AK, et al. Prevention of commotio cordis in baseball: an evaluation of chest protectors. *J. Trauma*. 2000; 49:1023-8.

[48] Weinstock J, Maron BJ, Song C, et al. Failure of commercially available chest wall protectors to prevent sudden cardiac death induced by chest wall blows in an experimental model of commotio cordis. *Pediatrics*. 2006; 117:656-62.

[49] Jackimczyk K. Blunt chest trauma. *Emerg. Med. Clin. North Am*. 1993; 11:81-96.

[50] Maron BJ, Gohman TE, Kyle SB, et al. Clinical profile and spectrum of commotio cordis. *JAMA*. 2002; 287:1142-6.

[51] Rodriguez A, Turney SZ. Blunt injuries of the heart and pericardium. In: Turney SZ, Rodriguez A, Cowley RA. Management of cardiothoracic trauma. Baltimore: *Williams & Wilkins*.1990; 261-84.

[52] Link MS, Estes NAM 3rd, Wang PJ, et al. Commotio cordis: cardiovascular manifestations of a rare survivor. *Chest*. 1998; 114:326-8.

[53] Marshall DT, Gilbert JD, Byard RW. The spectrum of findings in cases of sudden death due to blunt cardiac trauma-'commotio cordis'. *Am. J. Forensic. Med. Pathol*. 2008; 29:1-4.

[54] Miyazaki T, Ihama Y, Fuke C. An autopsy case of commotio cordis from a motor scooter accident. *Legal Med*. 2008; 10:264-7.

[55] Brugada P, Brugada J. Right bundle branch block, persistent ST segment elevation and sudden cardiac death: a distinct clinical and electrocardiographic syndrome: a multicenter report. *J. Am. Coll. Cardiol*. 1992; 20:1391-6.

[56] Maron BJ, Estes NA 3rd, Link MS. Task Force 11: Commotio cordis. *J. Am. Coll. Cardiol*. 2005; 45:1371-3.

[57] Osorio J, Dosdall DJ, Tabereaux PB, et al. Effect of chest compressions on ventricular activation. *Am. J. Cardiol*. 2012; 109:670-4.

[58] Maron BJ, Haas TS, Ahluwalia A, et al. Increasing survival rate from commotio cordis. *Heart Rhythm*. 2013; 10:219-23.

[59] Maron BJ, Strasburger JF, Kugler JD, et al. Survival following blunt chest impact-induced cardiac arrest during sports activities in young athletes. *Am. J. Cardiol*. 1997; 79:840-1.

[60] Cecchin F, Jorgenson DB, Berul CI, et al. Is arrhythmia detection by automated external defibrillator accurate for children?: sensitivity and specificity of an automated external defibrillator algorithm in 696 pediatric arrhythmias. *Circulation*. 2001; 103:2483-8.

[61] Guidelines 2000 for Cardiopulmonary Resuscitation and Emergency Cardiovascular Care. Part 4: The automated external defibrillator, key link in the chain of survival. *Circulation*. 2000; 102:I60-76.

[62] Carey CC, Callahan TJ. Automated external defibrillators in children: Food and Drug Administration Issues. In: Quan L, Franklin WH, et al. Ventricular Fibrillation: A Pediatric Problem. Armonk: *Futura Publishing Company*. 2000; 195-206.

[63] Janda DH, Viano DC, ANdrzejak DV, et al. An analysis of preventive methods for baseball-induced chest impact injuries. *Clin. J. Sport Med*. 1992; 2:172-9.

[64] Link MS, Bir C, Dau N, et al. Protecting our children from the consequences of chest blows on the playing field: a time for science over marketing. *Pediatrics*. 2008; 122:437-9.

[65] Van de Sandt F, Umans V. Acute cardiac events and deployment of emergency medical teams and automated external defibrillators in large football stadiums in the Netherlands. *Eur. J. Cardiovasc. Prev. Rehabil*. 2009; 16:571-5.

[66] Silka MJ, Bar-Cohen Y. Sudden cardiac death. In: Hugh DA. Moss and Adams' heart disease in infants, children, and adolescents. 7th Edition. Philadelphia: *Lippiocott Williams& Wilkins*. 2008; 356.

In: Rare Diseases
Editors: Giorgio Di Giovanni and Pietro Marcoz
ISBN: 978-1-62948-525-6

Chapter II

How to Develop a Comprehensive and Cross-Disease Approach to Improve Patients' Illness Experience and Meet Public Policy Makers' Expectations

Caroline Huyard*
Centre d'études et de recherches administratives,
Politiques et sociales (Ceraps)
Université Lille, Lille, France

Abstract

Rare diseases often have a negative impact on the personal, professional and social life of the patients. For this reason, taking into account both the medical and the social dimensions of the disease in patients' follow-up could improve patients' experience of the illness. However, implementing such a comprehensive approach can be difficult, because the related information, the skills or the temporal or material resources are not always available to medical teams.

One way to fill this gap is to work in partnership with the associations dedicated to rare disorders. Indeed, these associations gather a large proportion of patients. Even more numerous are the patients who only temporarily join in order to address a specific problem that the medical team had not been able to address directly or precisely. Some characteristics of these associations tend to affect the relationships with the medical teams who would be willing to set up a cooperation.

For this reason, it is useful to distinguish three different types of associations with respect to this potential cooperation. Finally, as there are many rare diseases, public

* E-mail: caroline.huyard@univ-lille2.fr.

policies targeting these conditions increasingly aim at taking an approach that address several rare diseases simultaneously.

One way to develop such a global approach is to focus on the issues that are common to several rare (and to some frequent) diseases. This issue-based approach is fortunately a key feature of the work carried out in some rare disease associations, and as such, it could be useful for medical teams wishing to develop the global, cross-disease vision that public policies are asking for.

Introduction

Rare diseases often have a negative impact on the personal, professional and social life of the patients (Van Nispen & Breuning 2003). As growing efforts are made to improve the situation of patients with rare diseases, identifying how the psycho-social issues could be best address would be useful.

On the one hand, implementing such a comprehensive approach can be difficult, because the related information, the skills or the temporal or material resources are not always available to medical teams.

On the other hand, the promotion of patients' autonomy, institutional reforms of the healthcare system that are aimed at improving users' participation, and patients' claims for the acknowledgement of their specific expertise, especially in the case of chronic illness, have contributed to the development of so-called "patients' organisations" (Wood 2000).

Some of these organisations have been very active in the medical and the public spheres, for instance through relationships with medical professionals (Bach 1998), action regarding biomedical research (Callon, Rabeharisoa 1999; Barbot 2002; Dalgalarrondo 2004; Epstein 2001; Novas 2005), or public health policy making (Wood 2000; Baggott, Allsop, Jones 2005).

Since the emergence of the category of "rare disorders", first in the Orphan Drug Act in the United States of America in the early 1980s, then in Japan, South Korea, Singapore, Taiwan and Australia in the 1990s, and in the Regulation on Orphan Medicinal Products of 2000 in the European Union, these associations have played a key role in improving patients' situation. In the United States of America, the National Organization for Rare Disorders was set up with the intention to educate the public and the medical community by acting as a clearing house of information on rare disorders.

In the European Union, patient representatives from rare disorder associations participate in the Committee for Orphan Medicinal Products, which reviews applications for the status of orphan medicinal products in Europe. In France, rare disorder associations number a total of 159 associations out of the 400 that were registered in 2013 by the *Institut National de la Santé et de la Recherche Médicale* (National Institute of Health and Medical Research) as being willing to support research projects. Thus, these organisations may provide some of the resources that medical staff need to address the psycho-social dimensions of rare disorders. Because of the historical and sociological use of the phrase "rare disorders", and not "rare diseases", these conditions will be termed "rare disorders" in this chapter.

However, commonly agreed definitions are still missing (Baggott, Forster 2008): they are usually referred to as "patients' associations" or "health consumer and patients' organisations", but as demonstrated by Chamak (2008), these terms do not apply in a number of cases, and especially when the organisations they relate to are actually "parents' organisations" and not "patients' organisations".

The classical issue of power within these particular organisations has been neglected, which is in line both with a lack of interest for the study of organisations in the field of medical sociology (that favoured social movements), and with a lack of interest for lay groups in health in the field of organisation studies (that investigated rather hospitals, clinics or health centres) (Davies 2003).

This is why a better understanding of these organisations is necessary. The purpose of this chapter is to answer three questions with respect to rare disorders associations and the needs of medical staff:

1. How important are rare disorders associations for the patients? These associations gather a large proportion of patients. Even more numerous are the patients who only temporarily join in order to address a specific problem that the medical team had not been able to address directly or precisely[1].
2. What are the characteristics of these associations that may affect the relationships with the medical teams who would be willing to set up a cooperation? Indeed, it is useful to distinguish three different types of associations with respect to this potential cooperation[2].
3. How could issues that are common to several rare disorders (and that are sometimes relevant to common diseases as well) be addressed? As there are many rare disorders, rare disorders public policies increasingly aim at taking an approach that address several rare disorders simultaneously. One way to develop such a global approach is to develop an issue-based approach. This is fortunately a key feature of the work carried out in some rare disorder associations, and as such, it could be useful for medical teams wishing to develop the global, cross-disease vision that public policies are asking for[3].

1. How Important Are Rare Disorders Associations for the Patients?

The overall aim of this part of the study is to identify the cause of patients' and their relatives' negative and positive judgements on the experience of a rare disorder, in order to establish to what extent the rarity of the disorder is an issue, by comparison with other characteristics (such as the genetic origin, the natural history of the disease, the lack of notoriety and the fear of an unknown disease, or the lack of institutional support through a specific organisation).

[1] This part draws on a previously published article: C. Huyard (2009) "What, if anything, is specific about having a rare disorder? Patients judgements on being ill and being rare", Health Expectations: an International Journal of Public Participation in Health Care and Health Policy, 12(4), 361-370.

[2] This part draws on a previously published article: C. Huyard (2009) "Who rules rare disease associations? A framework to understand their action", Sociology of Health and Illness, 31(7), 979-993.

[3] This part draws on a previously published book chapter: C. Huyard (2012) Rare. Sur la cause politique des maladies peu fréquentes, Paris, Editions de l'Ecole des Hautes Etudes en Sciences Sociales, chapter 7, p. 201-224.

The participants' judgements related to four themes: diagnosis, information, treatments and meeting other people with a rare condition. This research was conducted in France and empirically grounded on a sample of six rare disorders (i.e., whose prevalence is below 5/10,000 according to the European Regulation on Orphan Medicinal Products). The sample included cystic fibrosis, fragile X syndrome, Wilson's disease, mastocytosis, locked-in syndrome, and a syndrome that is especially infrequent, affecting only 5 persons in France, and that will be termed simply Very Rare Syndrome, in order to protect the confidentiality of the patients' identity and of their family.

Table 1. The six disorders and their characteristics

Characteristics of the diseases	Fragile X Syndrome	Cystic fibrosis	Wilson's disease	Mastocytosis	Locked-in syndrome	Very Rare Syndrome
Estimated number of affected persons in France	10,000	5,000	1,500	800	250	5
Origin	Genetic	Genetic	Genetic	Unknown	Accidental	Genetic
Typical age at presentation of the disease	Childhood	Childhood	Early adulthood	Any age	Adulthood	Childhood
Symptoms	Learning difficulties and behavioural troubles (shyness, autism)	Bronchial and rhinosinusal symptoms, pancreatic insufficiency and liver disease	Accumulation of copper in the body, with hepatic, neurologic or psychiatric presentation	Accumulation of mast cells in one or several organs	Complete paralysis, inability to speak, but fully preserved mental capabilities	Several organs are affected
Treatment	None	Symptomatic	Three different specific drugs	Symptomatic	None	Symptomatic
Impact on life-expectancy or current life-expectancy	None	40 years	None if treated adequately, a few months otherwise	Variable (lethal in 10% of the patients)	Variable	Variable
Notoriety	Weak	High: fund-raising campaigns	Weak	Weak	High: a book (Bauby 1997) has popularized the condition in France	None

The enquiry consists in 29 interviews with patients and 15 interviews with parents. These interviews were semi-structured, their average length was one hour, the same themes were covered in all cases, they were conducted by the same researcher, at the participants' home (for fragile X syndrome and the Very Rare Syndrome), at the hospital (for cystic fibrosis and

Wilson's disease) and at the association's seat (mastocytosis). Parents and patients were interviewed separately, except for three cases (two regarding Wilson's disease, one, the fragile X syndrome). Among the 29 patients, there were 15 women and 14 men, from 20 to 47 years old, 15 participants had cystic fibrosis, 10 had Wilson's disease, 3 had fragile X syndrome, and 1 had had mastocytosis. Among the 15 parents, there were only 3 fathers, 8 parents had at least one child with fragile X syndrome, 3 had at least one child with Wilson's disease, 2 had at least one child with cystic fibrosis, and 2 had one child with the Very Rare Syndrome. The diseases impacted the occupational status of the patients, whose distribution did not match that of the general population, whereas the occupational status of the parents did. In addition to the interview work, and with the organisers' approval, 15 meetings were attended within associations dedicated to rare disorders in general, to fragile X syndrome, to cystic fibrosis, to Wilson's disease and to locked-in syndrome, which allowed a more informal data collection, through informal talks with the participants. These talks covered the same themes as the interviews. They were subsequently transcribed, and compared with the data from the interviews.

The aspiration to meet other people with a rare disorder was massively shared by the participants, whatever their disease and its characteristics, genetic or not, curable or not. Thus, among the 10 participants with Wilson's disease, only 2 had never attended a national meeting of the corresponding association. Similarly, all the participants who have a child with fragile X syndrome are members of an association dedicated to the syndrome or, in only one case, to intellectual disability in general. According to the estimated prevalence reported in medical literature about the locked-in syndrome, mastocytosis and the Very Rare Syndrome, the corresponding associations were able to identify nearly all French patients. The case of cystic fibrosis is different, because the main association plays a key role in the organisation of care, making it difficult for patients to avoid contact with it. Besides, problems of cross-infections can arise when patients come together physically, which is a potential obstacle to such meetings.

The importance of the associative phenomenon was further analysed in the interviewees' discourse by combining two questions, in order to match the perception of having a rare feature with the relationships with others. Thus, the first question relates to the person's identity: to what extent is the fact of having a rare disorder perceived an important or, on the contrary, unimportant feature of one's identity? The answer to this question was provided by the way the participants depicted themselves and the following aspects: did they describe themselves as sick or very affected by the disease? Did they express the feeling of being different from others (e.g., a feeling of being displaced, being misunderstood, having particular features that are not shared outside the circle of those affected)? The second question relates directly to the relationships with others: what types of people does the participant aspire to meet? Does (s)he try to meet other people with the same disease or does (s)he try to avoid them?

The answers to these two questions resulted in four theoretical cases; 40 interviews were relevant in this regard (some participants insisted on their associative commitment rather than on their own experience, so the interviews did not provide enough information to determine which of the last two theoretical cases they matched):

1. the person does not wish to meet other people in the same situation and she does not view herself as having any rare feature,12 persons, patients and relatives.

2. the person does not wish to meet other people in the same situation and she views herself has rare in some regards, *no* participant matched this situation.
3. the person wishes to meet other persons in the same situation and she does not view herself as having any rare feature, 8 persons, mainly relatives.
4. the person wishes to meet other people in the same situation and she views herself has rare in some regards, 20 persons, relatives and patients.

Matching theoretical cases with empirical data suggests that it is extremely difficult both to feel rare and to remain isolated from other people with the same feature. None of the participants were in such a situation. This implies that, once illness has become an important aspect in the life of a person with a rare disorder, this person will try to meet other people with the same affection. When the disease is so rare that this is not possible, the person may try to meet people who also have a rare disorder, whatever it is. Within this inquiry, three persons in this situation were identified. Hoping to meet people who had an experience of rarity, they participated in an association dedicated to a rare disorder, although they did not have this particular disease. They were seeking answers to several moral questions: can they consider themselves as truly badly off? How to imagine a happy life with the disease? How to lead a good life, i.e., feeling useful and being cheerful? Thus, the encounter with people who have a disease that is medically very different remains meaningful, because the moral experience is similar enough.

These findings are coherent with many views the participants expressed about the role of associations. Thus, a participant with cystic fibrosis explained about the hypothetical future of the association, after the equally hypothetical discovery of a cure: "the association does not work so that (...) we can withdraw before the 'cure', in quotation marks, or before certain critical thresholds, when one would say, 'the association is not needed any more'. (...) And then, I think there is a comforting dimension, with the quality of life department, there will perhaps always be an association to provide hospitality, even if there are no more deaths…". Meeting other persons with the same rare specificity is crucial for the patients and their family, and a key feature of the rare disorder experience, whatever the characteristics of the diseases.

More so, rare disorders associations sometimes help the patients and their relatives, for instance in providing information that medical staff can hardly access. It is broadly admitted that medical knowledge is unsatisfactory for most rare disorders (Wolf 1994).

It appeared in the study that, if the patients were conscious that the progress of medical knowledge regarding their rare disorder should improve its treatment, medical knowledge was not their first concern.

They selected among the information they had been provided with what was most related to their daily life and their personal projects, and they quickly confused or forgot general information that they judged irrelevant in this regard. Their concern is mainly a moral one, i.e., it is related to their conception of what a good life is and of what the right way to behave is. Such questions are not easily answered by medical staff.

The participants' first aspiration was to be informed in order to be able to act in a way that allows them to reach their own goals. For this reason, the non-medical advice that health professionals provided them with often proved extremely helpful. This was the case at the time of diagnosis disclosure for a woman whose daughter has fragile X syndrome, as she explained: "I will always remember, my first question, our first question was, 'will she live?', because we had been told so many times that she probably had a serious illness.

It was our first question. (The physician) said 'yes, of course', so we thought, 'well, it's perfect'. And he said something else, that struck me, because our little girl was only six. He said, 'if your daughter reaches adulthood bearing in mind what she is, you will win'. This struck me."

The interviewee reported this advice was in her eyes the most valuable that a physician had given her regarding her daughter. Second, the patients' action-oriented perspective brings them and their relatives to view the disease according to a hierarchy in which abilities prevail over inabilities. This view stands in contradiction with the medical view, which is intrinsically based on deficiencies.

Many parents remembered that their first question at the time of the diagnosis had been "what will my child be able to do?". This perspective is not the one health professionals spontaneously adopt, although they could, as illustrated by the aforementioned example. Indeed, the physician provided the parents with a direction for their action, and this direction was based on a view of the child as able to achieve a specific attitude, not on deficiencies. On the contrary, these issues are typically the ones that are discussed by patients and their relatives during the meetings that rare disorders associations organise.

Information is merely one example among many others. Cooperating with these associations could help medical staff provide patients and their relatives the guidance they need for their daily life with the illness. This brings us to some questions regarding rare disorders associations for medical staff : what kind of organisations are they, what are the organisational characteristics that may foster or hamper cooperation, what are the roles that medical staff may play in these organisations ?

2. What Are the Characteristics of Rare Disorders Organisations That May Affect the Relationships with the Medical Teams Who Would Be Willing to Set up a Cooperation?

The aim of this part of the study is to describe the different types of rare disorders associations and how different stakeholders may be able to contribute within each type. A precise depiction of the inner structure of these associations, of their activities, of their goals and of the resources they tap into is needed to elaborate accurate distinctions between different types of organisation and thus better understand if a cooperation is possible and to what extent. The enquiry was conducted in France and empirically grounded on 8 organisations, matching the same 6 rare disorders as above.

On the basis of the empirical data on rare disorder associations presented here, I argue that the stakeholders' representation within the governing institution (e.g., Board of Directors) is decisive.

It has an impact on many other dimensions of the organisations, whatever the characteristics of the disease. Exploring the composition of rare disorder associations lead to identify two types of governing institution, whose description is the purpose of this study. Some governing institution bring together a broad array of different stakeholders who are willing to work together. This is why I suggest terming these organisations “pluralistic associations”.

In other governing institution, a single category of stakeholders firmly takes the lead and strives to control the actions of the other, subordinate, stakeholders. With respect to the “pluralistic associations” those are a contrast to, I suggest calling them “monistic associations”. Among these monistic associations, a further distinction is to be made between those that have only little financial resources ("recognition-claiming associations"), and those that have much more of it ("radical associations").

Table 2. The 8 associations and the characteristics of their structure

Organisations	Related condition	Year of creation	Founders	Rough annual budget	Mains sources of funding
Le Goéland (Seagull)	Fragile X Syndrome	1991	A couple of parents	Less than one hundred thousands euros	Occasional sponsorships and subsidies
Mosaïques (Mosaics)	Fragile X Syndrome	1993	A mother	Less than one hundred thousands euros	Memberships
Vaincre la Mucoviscidose (Defeating Cystic Fibrosis)	Cystic Fibrosis	1965	Physicians and parents	Millions of euros	Regular fund-raising campaigns; sponsorships
ABCF Mucoviscidose (ABCF Cystic Fibrosis)	Cystic Fibrosis	1998	One physician	Hundreds of thousands of euros	Sponsorships and donations
Association Bernard Pépin pour la maladie de Wison (Bernard Pépin Association for Wilson's Disease)	Wilson's disease	1989	Physicians, patients and relatives	Tens of thousands of euros	Donations; occasional sponsorships
Afirmm: Association française pour les initiatives de recherche sur le mastocyte et les mastocytoses (French Association for research initiatives on mastocyte and mastocytosis)	Mastocytosis	1999	One lay person	Millions of euros	A proportion of the related biotech firm's benefits
Alis: Association du Locked-in Syndrome (Locked-in Syndrome Association)	Locked-in Syndrome	1997	One patient (author of a best-seller about this condition) and one health professional	Less than one hundred thousands euros	Donations and subsidies
Very Rare Syndrome Association	Very Rare Syndrome	After 2000	A couple of parents	None	None

Pluralistic Associations

There were three "pluralistic associations" in the sample: *Vaincre la mucoviscidose*, the *Association Bernard Pépin pour la maladie de Wilson* and the *Association du locked-in syndrome*. They cover a range of diseases with different characteristics, since they represent two genetic diseases (one disease that remains incurable and lethal, and a disease whose natural history is also lethal but can generally be efficiently reversed) and one non-genetic disability. These organizations are characterized primarily by the fact that they bring together patients, their relatives and health professionals, all of them as equals and fully requested in the association's governing body. Their action covers a temporal scope that includes both the near and the distant future, and does not rely on the expectation of a medical breakthrough that would dramatically alter its goals.

The willingness to gather different stakeholders has been present since the creation of these organisations, whatever the date of their creation (in the 1960s, the 1980s or the 1990s), and it has remained the main drive for all the participants. Indeed the goals that these associations had given themselves in their early days tightly depended upon such a grouping: they deemed it necessary to gain public health administration's official acknowledgement of the disease for the one[4], to end the patients' isolation for the other[5], and to provide both health professionals, patients and families with emotional and material support for the third one[6]. The achievement of each of these goals implied assembling as many people as possible. The three associations have been created jointly by health professionals and by "lay" persons, and more precisely, by clinicians and patients in two cases, and by clinicians and parents in one case, the patients themselves joining the organisation later, when their increased life expectancy and number allowed them to get involved.

The board of directors of each of these associations includes three categories of stakeholders: (1) health professionals, (2) patients, (3) relatives of the patients, with the first category on the one hand and the second and the third categories on the other hand roughly on an equal numerical footing. In two cases, health professionals were in the majority when the organisation was founded[7]. Health professionals frequently are clinical investigators, i.e., professionals who work both as care providers and as researchers. In all cases, an effort is made to include in the permanent structures of the association representatives of all the professionals who face the disease, including paramedical professions[8]. The internal organisation of these associations displays some slight differences. Thus, two out of the three associations have a scientific board. In one case, it has remained inactive since the creation of the association, because the association focussed on care and social support and planned no research project. In the other, it is but one board among others (medical board, patients' board, associative life board). Most of these boards are made up of one category of stakeholders only, although they regularly have work sessions with external experts who do not belong to this category. In the third association, health professionals who often were already active members of the main association have created a specific independent association that brings

---

[4] Interviews with founding physicians (5 May 2004, 18 June 2004) and a founding parent (April 2003)

[5] Interview with an employee (3 June 2004)

[6] Interview with a physician (14 March 2005)

[7] Interviews with physicians (18 June 2004, 14 March 2005) and a parent (April 2003)

[8] Interviews with an employee (3 June 2004), physicians (17 January 2005, 14 March 2005) and a parent (14 October 2004)

together clinician-investigators who have an interest in the disease[9]. Both this scientific council and the independent association are designed to foster the exchange and the progress of knowledge, in different and evolving ways (Larédo, Kahane 1998). But this is not true of all entities referred to as a "scientific board", as we shall see later on.

The members of these associations do not consider their collective action as having a definite end time. This is not a surprise in the case of locked-in syndrome, since it is viewed as a disability that is unlikely to be cured, but that rather demands ongoing efforts towards the patients' integration. On the contrary, the case of Wilson's disease is especially illuminating in this respect, since the association tends to be increasingly active, although very effective treatments have been available for decades. The case of cystic fibrosis is different insofar as it remains a life-shortening disease with symptomatic treatment, but the participants insisted they were engaged in a lengthy process that is not intended to come to its end with the hypothetical discovery of an efficient therapy.

Collective action encompasses a broad temporal scope that implies the collaboration of different stakeholders, be they those who have a concern for the present or those who care for the distant future. The series of presentations of the association's activities, at the general assembly of one of the "pluralistic associations", illustrates this point: a biologist discussed the patients' diet on the basis of a nutrition book that a family had given to the association, a neurologist presented the preliminary results of an ongoing research on pregnancy for the patients on the basis of a questionnaire that was filled in by members of the association, and then discussed the future creation of a European database of the patients, a project supported by public organisations, a pharmaceutical company and corresponding disease associations[10]. Another association allocates 30% of its financial means to biomedical research projects, 20% to healthcare improvement, 10% to social assistance, and 15% to information campaigns[11]. Another one offers emotional and practical support by telephone, creates videotapes to educate health professionals, and maintains relationships with different healthcare institutions in order to educate them, help them to improve the quality of their services, and lobby for the patients[12].

In spite of major differences between the three conditions that the "pluralistic associations" are dedicated to, the organisations themselves display many similarities regarding their respective actions. This suggests that medical issues are not key to understanding the way rare disorder associations operate. On the contrary, political issues (i.e., how the stakeholders consider collective action and take part in it), especially the composition of the organisation, seem decisive. The comparison with the other type of association, namely "monistic associations", provides further evidence.

Monistic Associations

A single category of stakeholders runs "monistic associations". These organisations may include categories other than the leading one, but those will then stand in a subordinate position, typically acting as advisers that do not actually take part in the decisions. This

[9] Interview with a physician (14 March 2005)
[10] General Assembly (12 March 2005)
[11] Association's activity reports.
[12] Interview with an employee (3 June 2004).

particular composition and distribution of power shapes collective relationships that are very different from those of "pluralistic associations". Notably, (1) there are no collaborative relationships, i.e., relationships between equals who share a common goal, but rather attempts to turn the participation of non-leading stakeholders into means to an end, and (2) these organisations consider their action as having a definite end time that would be achieved through a "revolutionary", i.e., sudden and deep, change, and that may justify neglecting other, more immediate, goals. However, this group of "monistic organisations" is not as homogeneous as the pluralistic ones, and it is necessary to distinguish two different types of "monistic associations" according to whether they have financial means at their disposal. I suggest terming the "monistic associations" that have very little means "recognition-claiming associations", and those that have financial means that enable them to take independent and potentially effective action "radical associations". I shall explain why hereafter.

The "recognition-claiming monistic associations" are the two associations dedicated to fragile X syndrome and the one dedicated to the Very Rare Syndrome. They have only little financial means (i.e., some meetings are cancelled or postponed because they cannot be funded, the association's representatives sometimes use their own private resources to carry out actions, and long- or medium-term actions are hardly planned). They can be viewed as recognition-claiming for several reasons. Their concrete action mainly aims at insisting that they and the disease that they represent exist and deserve attention. Thus, the actions of these organisations vary little over time, and identical projects are continued without any assessment or amendment, with the idea that they will contribute towards publicizing their cause. The scientific board, when there is one, mostly serves as a support for the association's credibility. Finally, if the associations' representatives often insist that they act in partnership with health professionals, this partnership is much more an aspiration than a reality, and the leading stakeholders actually take action on their own. The association of the Very Rare Syndrome being more recent and particularly small, the other two associations will be the focus of this section.

The associations *Le Goéland* and *Mosaïques* were created respectively by a couple of parents and by a mother, with the support of one or two health professionals who do not have any responsibilities within the associations, and are sometimes not even members of them[13]. These organisations consider themselves to be parents' associations. The board of directors is exclusively made up of parents. Fifteen years after the creation of these organisations, the founders still play a key role and remain in the same positions. Actually, their original view of collective action is very different from the one of the "pluralistic associations". The association is above all considered as a means "to be heard, to be acknowledged, and to be supported"[14], not as a working platform for several categories of stakeholders. It is a tool for demanding assistance from other potential stakeholders, not for creating the means of mutual exchange. This goal tends to be the main one of these associations.

What feelings or objectives drive these associations' representatives is an issue that deserves attention. Commitment is described as an authentic emotional and moral need. How powerful it is, is clearly expressed by an association's representative: "We were sort of enraged. And when we stopped working on information, on training and all that, if we were no longer working for that, we became sick". Some parents even come to consider

---

[13] Interviews with parents (6 July 2004, 5 January 2005)

[14] Interview with a parent (6 July 2004)

substituting for health professionals, as a mother explains: "I even thought of resuming studies in biochemistry, in order to really understand, and to do research". These attitudes can be viewed as two different ways for individuals to become overwhelmed by the action against the disease, in the first case because this action has turned out to be a vital need, and in the second one because it changes one's status from that of parent to one of health professional. Moreover, the motivations of these associations' leaders make it extremely difficult for them to delegate power, since the boundaries between themselves and the rest of the association are blurred. This has many consequences for these organisations, which challenge the emergence of an authentic collective.

The scientific board in such associations greatly differs from that of "pluralistic associations". Two of the recognition-claiming associations have such a board. It is not a platform for a common dynamic, its members hardly have meetings[15], but they are expected to guarantee the credibility of the organisation, by accepting to have their names mentioned in relation to it, and by providing medical or scientific information when needed. Besides, the composition of this council reflects that the association's leaders have a restrictive view of the relevant stakeholders. If they aspire to have researchers and medical doctors join their organisation, they consider neither the participation of the patients themselves, nor that of care or social work professionals. This is a contrast to the inclusive approach of the "pluralistic associations". Thus, the patients who might participate perceive the association as their parents', and not as a group to which they could participate[16].

The temporal scope of collective action is not defined in a collective way within these organisations. On the one hand, it is closely influenced by the past experience or by the present difficulties of the founders themselves, and is not necessarily related to the most important issues for all the associations' members. Thus, during the 1980s, the founding families confronted health professionals, notably psychiatrists, being hardly aware of the genetic component of certain intellectual conditions, and they have subsequently devoted a great effort to the organization of symposia, in 1995 and 2000, aimed at getting these professionals to open up to genetics. However, associations do not attempt to assess the impact of these events, therefore repeating them over time, and they tend to neglect other issues, such as securing the future of the children with an intellectual disability after the death of their parents, although all the interviewees with children with the fragile X syndrome said that this is one of their major worries. On the other hand, the associations insist on the idea that collective action will eventually end, thanks to "revolutionary" medical discoveries. Thus, each time research results are published, the associations' leaders expect the imminence of major changes, as illustrated by this comment from an association's representative: "from there (the understanding of one mechanism involved in the disease), everything will explode, we will be given all the means, the laboratories will look at us". Ordinary members have an ambiguous attitude towards this view. They appreciate it, because they believe it "brings hope"[17], but they also admit that they actually expect no such breakthrough, and merely desire better care here and now for their children.

Lastly, the actual collaboration between these associations and health professionals is poor. Since 2004 in France, specific hospital units for rare disorders have been granted a

[15] Interview with a physician (7 January 2005)
[16] Interviews with patients (19 January 2005, 11 March 2005)
[17] Informal discussions at the General Assembly (6-8 May 2005)

nationwide specific designation, as reference centres, which acknowledges their expertise and improves their funding. The units that planned to apply for reference centre status solicited the "pluralistic associations" (in which some of their members were often already committed) to gain their support[18]. Some associations had even fostered the creation of similar units before the national movement was launched[19]. But there has been no similar dynamic of cooperation in the case of these recognition-claiming associations[20]. Similarly, as an association representative reported, the disagreement between the mean age at the time of the diagnosis measured by one association and that measured by the laboratories that perform the diagnosis reflects how difficult it is to work together: "I had written that the mean age at the time of the diagnosis is three years old and we can be proud of it... And my geneticist called me, telling me, 'the eighteen laboratories in France who are interested in the fragile X have calculated an average age, and indeed the mean age at the time of the diagnosis is 11.6 years.' So it means that there are huge regional disparities."

These associations are a contrast to "pluralistic associations" in many ways: the willingness to be supported is greater than that to engage in a collective work with other groups, and especially with a scientific board; action is highly emotion-driven, as opposed to the collaboration-driven action of "pluralistic associations", its temporal scope is strongly influenced both by past experience and the way the leaders picture an ideal future and tends to neglect the present or the near future; and a sudden "back to normalcy" state is hoped for, which is considered a nonsense in "pluralistic associations". Associations that have a similar monistic composition but also financial means to carry out actions display features that are just as opposed to those of "pluralistic associations", but in slightly different ways.

The two other "monistic associations", namely *ABCF Mucoviscidose* and *Afirmm,* have also set themselves one objective and consider that the other stakeholders should assist them with its fulfilment, but what is more, they have secured the financial means to reach their goal (through annual budgets that are above one hundred thousand euros and up to millions of euros). They both display the characteristics of what Simmel (1902) has identified as being small groups' "sociological radicalism": "it is marked by the unreserved dedication of the individual to the tendency of the group, by the sharp delimitation of the same against neighbouring structures which is necessary to the self-preservation of the group, by the impossibility of taking up into the externally narrow frame a multitude of far-reaching endeavours and thoughts" (p 9). The first characteristic is doubly present in this case, both with individual aspirations being completely subordinated to the collective goal and with the hegemony of a single person on the whole organisation. The second characteristic takes the form of a relentless condemnation of the strategic choices of the other associations in the field. Finally, these associations pursue over the years a single objective, without deviating from it or critically reviewing it. I argue that this radicalism results both from the monistic structure of the organisation and from the importance of its financial resources.

Both "monistic radical associations" were created by one person who still has the lead, a medical doctor in one case, a lay person in the other. Both pursue a single goal, respectively to support research projects on pharmacological treatments of CF with a focus on the role of proteins and to find a cure for mastocytosis. Both associations have a scientific board that

---

[18] General Assembly (12 March 2005)
[19] Interview with a parent (7 March 2003)
[20] General Assembly (6-8 May 2005)

validates the scientific orientations of the association, whereas, in "pluralistic associations", schematically, the board of directors validates the orientations of the scientific board. Thus, "collective" action is monitored by a single category of stakeholders or a single person and strives for a single aim (however, this aim varies from one association to the other). As an association's representative explained: "We have put in the mission of the association to cure the disease. And that's that. I refused systematically all the social tasks of an association. There is no social mission. I never speak to patients, well I speak, but it is to develop a trial, this sort of thing. But there are no welfare activities. People would say, 'but we wanted to be able to talk with people with this disease', and we answer, 'no'. Or rather, we don't say no, we say, 'that's your problem!'[21] Lastly, an important feature of these associations' discourse is their contrasting of a dark past with a bright future, as in this information leaflet on cystic fibrosis: "the gene of cystic fibrosis was discovered in 1989, 19 years ago. For 19 years, parents have hoped, and patients have tried to wait. During these 19 years, some were unable to wait, and others will soon not be able to wait any more. (...) Today, we cannot cure cystic fibrosis. What we can do tomorrow is up to you".

Recognition-claiming associations and radical associations thus do not only differ with respect to their means, but display a series of disparities: the first ones strive to be heard, the second strive to take action; the recognition-claiming association's leaders tend to be emotionally overwhelmed by their cause and struggle to keep the organisation going, whereas those in radical associations firmly control the organisation's action; the scientific board serves as a credential provider in one case, and as a means to an end in the other; there is thus nearly no collaboration at all in recognition-claiming associations whereas collaboration is an instrument to achieve a self-set and self-monitored goal in radical associations. However, both types of "monistic associations" share a specific temporal scope that tends to insist that the future is more important than the present. This stance does not favour critically assessing the actions that have been taken, but rather rushing in. An important question then is that of the dynamic relationships between these two types of "monistic associations": what are the paths that lead from one to the other? What about "pluralistic organisations"?

From Recognition-Claiming to Radical Associations

Considering the descriptions of rare disorder associations in a number of studies (Wexler 1996; Bach 1998; Callon, Rabeharisoa 1999; Stockdale 1999; Novas 2005), it seems that a radical association is the type of organization that has elicited the greatest scholarly interest. In France, the French Muscular Dystrophy Association (AFM) has thus been the subject of several studies (Paterson, Barral 1994; Bach 1998; Callon, Rabeharisoa 1999; Rabeharisoa 2003). These studies allow one to say that this is an association of parents, who make decisions on their own, even if they take the advice of a scientific council, and whose goal is primarily the funding of scientific research. Bach's very detailed history of the relationships between lay people and biomedical professionals within the AFM (1998) suggests that the transition from a recognition-claiming association to a radical one was made possible by the unexpected success of the first large-scale television-based fund-raising campaign of 1987. Thus, Bach quotes the former AFM president, who declared after this first fund-raising event:

[21] Interview (30 June 2004)

"the situation is radically different: before, we could only ask, without offering in return. Since December, 6, the balance of power has shifted" (p 252).

Thus, the key difference between mere recognition-claiming associations and radical associations may not be found in the leading category of stakeholders, since this may be parents (AFM), health professionals (*ABCF Mucoviscidose*) or others (Afirmm), with different goals in each case (research in general, or a specific area of research, or the development of a potential cure). It does not seem to result from the specific characteristics of the disease, as both recognition-claiming and radical organisations include genetic (notably CF and muscular dystrophies) and non-genetic diseases (mastocytosis), and very different types of organisations (pluralistic as well as radical) may match the same disease (CF). Rather, it is the access to financial resources that seems to induce the shift from one type to the other. Regarding "pluralistic associations", the history of those studied here suggests they may turn into monistic ones, generally after a group split from the original organisation, but the contrary does not seem to have happened.

A common underlying assumption in "patient" organisations studies is that it is necessary to revert the balance of power present in the therapeutic relationships by providing lay people with a decision monopoly within these associations. But this focus on the therapeutic relationships at the expense of consideration of the diversity of stakeholders appears as being inappropriate. Indeed, as a now classical study in organisation theory (Armstrong 1977) demonstrated, through the thorough analysis of a role playing case, stakeholder diversity is a powerful means to achieve social responsibility regarding corporate governance: whereas 79% of the role playing groups that represented only one category of actors, namely stockholders, took socially harmful decisions, this was only the case of 22% of the groups that represented a broad range of diverse stakeholders. The results presented here are in line with this study.

This suggests that, in a normative perspective, and contrary to what is often assumed, "pluralistic organisations" are likely to perform better. This would deserve further studies. The interviewees in "recognition claiming monistic associations" generally expressed their desire to see their organisation evolving into a pluralistic one, and the possibility of such an evolution is an issue for investigation, since it did not appear in this study. On the contrary, several "recognition claiming monistic associations" were created by people who had broken away from a "pluralistic organisation". The interviewees in "radical monistic associations" had no such critical look on their organisation. This points to the important question of the options that are available for the stakeholders who do not have the lead in these associations, and seem to choose "loyalty" rather than "voice" or "exit" (Hirschman 1972).

3. How Could Issues That Are Common to Several Rare (and Frequent) Disorders Be Addressed?

A the level of each rare disorder organisation, the desire to put an end to isolation is often the first step towards the group, but it is not what makes people stay with the group, neither what grounds the organisation. Within the organisation, people are together because they consider a common issue, and wish to work on this issue in a collective way. rare disorder organisations typically strive to identify patients, offer training for health care providers, or raise awareness about their cause. For each of these tasks, the contribution of many different actors is very helpful. These actors do need specific competences (regarding medical knowledge, communication skills, fundraising skills...) and they do not particularly need to be directly affected by the condition. These organisations can be termed issue-based: people come together to struggle with a range of problems that they want to solve. The relationships *between* such rare disorder organisations are not issue-based, and they tend to be rarity-based.

This part of the study draws on 27 interviews with patients and relatives who found the topic of collective action relevant, and who discussed the Telethon (the major fundraising event for a rare disorders in France), rare disorders coalitions and coalition work, and the goals and functions of the association dedicated to their own rare disorder. The organisations come together because their members address rare disorders. How this should work exactly was not clear for the persons I have interviewed as members of a rare disorder organisation. The interviewees considered three principles: one for all, each one should care for themselves, all for one.

According to the "one for all" principle, solidarity between rare disorders organisations is based on the idea that any advancement for one disorder will benefit many other disorders. The interviewees who support this view do so with great conviction, but they are not the majority, being in a proportion of only one out of three respondents. They tend to say that they actually expect little medical progress, and that they are not hoping for a cure for themselves. One of the participants in the study, a women with Wilson's disease explained for instance:

> Question: what would you like your association to undertake?
>
> Answer: supporting research. It is true that there are not so many of us, but we could imagine taking actions that would yield money for research, but not necessarily *our* money, we could think of actions that could... Well, it seems we are not so badly off [...] and it seems that they use the money that comes from the Telethon to fund a little research... And anyway, the research that is carried out for orphan diseases bring advances for diseases such as Wilson's disease. [her emphasis]

According to the "each one should care for themselves" principle, solidarity between rare disorders organisations does not make much sense. For the majority of the interviewees (two out of 3 respondents), it is paramount to support one's own rare disorder organisation, although they were always very embarrassed to express this view. In some cases these interviewees had first supported the "one for all" view, but were disappointed, and changed their mind. Most of the respondents said they viewed the "each one should care for themselves" principle as more pragmatic, more effective, while being more selfish, and morally inferior.

One of the participant, a man with Wilson's disease explained for instance:

> I have never given any money to the Telethon. It's probably a bit selfish but I have never watched the Telethon. [...]
>
> You do not feel concerned

> I cannot say I'm not concerned, but... I'm not interested. Well, yes, I don't feel I'm concerned. I think... It's selfish, but the problem is that... It's not focused. If it had focussed on Wilsons disease, I would have watched. It's a selfish view. I don't care about the other genetic disorders. I care about the one I have, not about the others.
>
> I have met many people who said they prefer giving to their association (he starts speaking again)
>
> Yes, because the actions are scattering. They are scattering, there is no clear direction. I prefer giving to the association [for Wilson's disease] that to the Telethon. Actually, the Telethon, it's for people who are not ill!
>
> What do you mean?
>
> Well, the people who give.
>
> Right, you mean that someone who is not ill has no particular concern for one disease, and will be able to give for something that is not focussed?
>
> Yes.

According to the "all for one" principle, solidarity is moral, and should not be considered in such a pragmatic way. Only two interviewees supported this view, that is a bit more complicated than the first two. It separates medical aspects from moral aspects. On a medical plane, these interviewees view all rare disorders as very different, and eliciting different expectations and goals. On a moral plane, these interviewees believe that the difficulties are however very similar, and that any progress for one single person should be seen as benefiting directly all the patients with a rare disorder. A woman whose son has Wilson's disease said for instance :

> Question: do you watch the Telethon ?
>
> Answer : a little, a little, not much. But I have notice that there were a sign for Wilson's disease this year, among the other diseases ! After the demonstration, when the people who had demonstrated had just arrived, they interviewed someone, and then, I've seen the sign "Wilson's disease". It was really very close, so I have seen it without looking for it. But otherwise, I don't look for it. But I was pleased. I was pleased to see that the association had joined the rare disorders associations. Because I feel sorry for all the other rare disorders. It's hard for Philip [her son], but some other diseases are really awful too.

All three principles bring difficulties. It is very clear that the "each one should care for themselves" principle creates no solidarity, and may reinforce competition between rare disorders organisations. The "one for all" principle, although it may seem less selfish, does not create more solidarity, because each organisation is in a way also waiting for their own benefit. The "all for one" principle tends to create more solidarity, but it is morally very demanding, and does not say anything about the way common work should be organised in practice.

Within each one of the rare disorders association, what grounds collective action is a range of issues (Dewey, 2003). People join together because of a common issue that they want to address together. For instance, in order to identify the patients, to train healthcare workers for specific tasks, to provide information on the disease to the patients and their relatives, or to raise awareness the associations need a range of competences from a range of different people, and focus on these competences. The people involved may be directly affected by the disease, but it is not considered important.

This is apparent when rare disorders associations work together with common disorders associations. These cooperations are based on the issue principle: these associations are addressing a common problem, and do not consider the number of patients as relevant. For instance, the cystic fibrosis association was involved in projects regarding patient's professional difficulties and was working with cancer associations and AIDS associations on the topic of evolving health conditions in the workplace. Similarly, the locked-in syndrome association, a tiny organisation, was working on home care issues with the big French associations that are dedicated to physical disabilities and run residential centres ; one of the fragile X syndrome associations had the same purpose with the associations dedicated to intellectual disabilities. In these cases, cooperation is based on complementarity and subsidiarity on particular issues, and not on diseases prevalence.

Discussion and Conclusion

The results presented here draw on a study that had three main limitations. First, it was limited to the French case. Second, it aimed at covering the widest possible diversity of diseases in a small sample, although rare disorders are very heterogeneous and very numerous. In particular, some characteristics of the diseases may be important, and in particular, the outcomes of this study may mostly apply to chronic rare disorders, whereas acute rare disorders would present a different picture. Third, it was limited to nationwide organizations, which excludes a myriad of local associations, and in particular associations which act as service providers in a definite geographic area. There is a need for more international and comparative research, including studies that look simultaneously at rare and frequent disorders, to overcome these limitations. Yet, for practitioners, this study yielded interesting hints for the improvement of patient's care.

The issues that patients mentioned suggests that cooperations between health professionals and rare disorders organisations may help better address important but still somewhat neglected needs. The participants voiced their need for disease-related associations. This is a key feature of rare disorder experience, that may result from the diseases' rarity and the feelings of isolation, invisibility and powerlessness it breeds. This was apparent in the case of information needs. The participants said they wished to be provided with appropriate guidance and not mere knowledge. The lack of medical information may thus be mitigated by less medical but not less adequate, comforting and action-supporting moral advice regarding daily life. This type information is generally not available to health professionals, but rather to more experienced patients themselves.

Cooperation of health professionals will be easier and more effective with organisations that have an adequate composition of their governing institutions. Indeed, if the therapeutic relationship is simple and asymmetrical, a whole organization dedicated to a disease includes a set of relationships that is totally different, broader and more complex. It is therefore important to adopt a view of mutual relationships that is adapted to collective action when studying it, and that does not draw on the model of therapeutic relationships. This study highlighted that is not so much the patient/doctor or lay/expert opposition that determines the operations of rare disorder associations than the composition of the leading group, a leadership shared between several categories of stakeholders being in contrast to a leadership exerted by a single stakeholder category, whatever this one is. The former organisations will be more willing to cooperate and target a range of different goals and dimensions of illness than the latter.

Cooperation will also be easier with organisations that have adopted an issue-based approach. As the need for overcoming the limitations of the "all for one" and "each one should care for themselves" principles in the design of dedicated healthcare centres, in research projects and within coalitions of rare disorders organisations, some insights from the political science literature on associations working together as a group are particularly relevant for a comprehensive and cross-disease approach :

- Coalitions are relevant when they are formed for a specific purpose and when they remain temporary (Lemieux, 1998). That's typically what happened with the Orphan Drug Act or with the European regulation on orphan medicinal products.
- Within a group of associations, it may be helpful to organize "issue-based" sub-groups, that is, sub-groups dedicated to different practical issues (Couto, 1998). For instance, issues regarding access to insurance or discrimination in the workplace, if these problems are common to a range of different disorders (that do not need to be unfrequent, such as aids, cancer or cystic fibrosis).
- It is important to ensure consistency between the organizational principles of individual associations and those of their federation (Couto, 1998). This suggests for instance that Europe-wide federation of associations of the same rare disorder could draw on existing "issue-based" national organisations to spread as a federation.
- The benefit that each association withdraws from participating in the group must be taken into account, because there is otherwise a risk that the "each one should care for themselves" strategy seems more attractive (Hojnacki, 1997). This point was very clear with the interviewees who thought that their organisation would benefit from joining others, and were disappointed afterwards.

REFERENCES

Armstrong J. S. (1977) "Social irresponsibility in management", *Journal of Business Research*, 5(3), 185-213.

Bach M.-A. (1998) "Building the French Muscular Dystrophy Association: the role of doctor/patient interactions", *Social History of Medicine*, 11(2), 233-253.

Baggott, R., Allsop, J., J& ones K. (2005) Speaking for Patients and Carers: Health Consumer Groups and the Policy Process, Basingstoke: Palgrave.

Baggott, R., & Forster, R. (2008) "Health consumer and patients' organizations in Europe: towards a comparative analysis", *Health Expectations*, 11, 85-94.

Barbot, J. (2002) Les malades en mouvement, la médecine et la science à l'épreuve du sida, Paris : Balland;

Bauby, J.-D. (1997) Le Scaphandre et le Papillon, Paris : Robert Laffont.

Callon, M., & Rabeharisoa, V. (1999), Le pouvoir des malades, l'association française contre les myopathies et la recherche, Paris: Presses de l'Ecole des Mines.

Chamak, B. (2008) "Autism and social movements: French parents' associations and international autistic individuals' organisations", *Sociology of Health and Illness*, 30(1):76-96.

Couto R. (1998) "Community coalitions and grassroots policies of empowerment", *Administration and Society*, 30(5), 569-574.

Dalgalarrondo, S. (2004) Sida: la course aux molécules, Paris : Editions de l'E.H.E.S.S.

Davies C. (2003) "Some of our concepts are missing: reflections on the absence of a sociology of organisations in Sociology of Health and Illness", *Sociology of Health and Illness*, 25 172-190.

Dewey J. (2003) Le public et ses problèmes, Pau/Tours/Paris: Publications de l'université de Pau/Farrago/Léo Scheer.

Epstein S. (2001) Histoire du sida, Paris: Les empêcheurs de penser en rond.

Hirschman A.O. (1972) Face au déclin des entreprises et des institutions, Paris: Economie et humanisme.

Hojnacki M. (1997) "Interest groups' decision to join alliances or work alone", *American Journal of Political Science*, 41(1), 61-87.

Larédo, P., & Kahane, B. (1998) "Politique de recherche et choix organisationnels de l'Association française de lutte contre la mucoviscidose", Sciences Sociales et Santé, 16(3), 97-126.

Lemieux V. (1998) Les coalitions. Liens, transactions et contrôles, Paris: PUF.

Novas C. (2005) "Genetic advocacy groups, science and biovalue: creating political economies of hope" in New genetics, new identities, .Atkinson, P.; Glasner, P. (ed.), London: Routledge.

Paterson, F., & Barral C. (1994) "L'A.F.M.: trajectoire d'une association d'usagers et construction associative d'une maladie", *Sciences Sociales et Santé*, 12(2), 79-111.

Rabeharisoa, V. (2003) "The struggle against neuromuscular diseases in France and the emergence of a 'partnership model' of patient organisation", Social Science and Medicine, 57, 2127-2136.

Simmel, G. (1902) "The Number of Members as Determining the Sociological Form of the Group: I." *American Journal of Sociology*, 8, 1-46.

Stockdale, A. (1999). Waiting for the cure: mapping the social relations of human gene therapy research, *Sociology of Health and Illness,* 21(5) 579-596.

Van Nispen, R.M.A., & Breuning, E. (2003). Rare diseases, a bibliography on health care and daily life, Netherlands Institute for Health Services Research: Utrecht.

Wexler, A. (1996) Mapping fate, a memoir of family, risk and genetic research, Berkeley: University of California Press.

Wolf A. (1994) Les orphelins de la santé. Paris: Editions Inserm.

Wood, B. (2000) Patient Power? The Politics of Patients' Associations in Britain and America, Buckingham & Philadelphia: Open University Press.

In: Rare Diseases
Editors: Giorgio Di Giovanni and Pietro Marcoz
ISBN: 978-1-62948-525-6

Chapter III

MuSK Myasthenia - A Rare Variant of a Rare Disease: A Case Description and Review of the Medical Literature

Michal Haran[1], Andras Mate[2], Daniel Starobin[3], Gregory Papirov[4] and Ami Schattner[5]
[1]Hematology Institute, Kaplan Medical Center, Rehovot, Israel
[2]Neurology unit, Kaplan Medical Center, Rehovot, Israel
[3]Pulmonology Unit, Kaplan Medical Center, Rehovot, Israel
[4]Respiratory long term care, Beit Rivka, Petach Tikva, Israel
[5]Department of Internal medicine A,
Kaplan Medical Center, Rehovot, Israel

Abstract

Muscle-specific kinase (MuSK) myasthenia gravis (MG) is a relatively rare autoimmune disease. Although it shares many features with the more common form of autoimmune myasthenia, i.e., acetylcholine receptor (AChR)-positive, there are many differences in the clinical manifestations, pathophysiology and response to treatment. This leads to significant difficulties in the diagnosis and management of this illness.

Whereas the function of the AChR is well understood, this is not so regarding MuSK. Little is known about the roles of this complex protein. In the embryonic period it is essential for proper assembly of the neuromuscular junction, but emerging evidence suggests that it may have other roles as well.

Conflicting data obtained from different patient groups and experimental models suggest that anti-MuSK antibodies are not uniform, and therefore exert a different effect depending on the epitope they are directed to.

Furthermore, most of the data in the medical literature is based on patients who have evidence for neuromuscular transmission defects. Yet, there are sporadic descriptions and case reports which suggest that other mechanisms may be at play.

This chapter will describe a case of a patient with MuSK MG; review the current knowledge regarding MuSK and MuSK MG while postulating possible mechanisms and suggesting better ways to diagnose this illness based on its unique pathophysiology, as well as areas for further clinical and basic research.

Introduction

The existence of a muscle-specific kinase (MuSK) variant of autoimmune myasthenia gravis (MG), a disease classically associated with anti-acetylcholine receptor (AChR) antibodies, was first suggested over a decade ago, when antibodies targeting MuSK were found in a subgroup of patients with seronegative MG [1]. However, the pathogenicity of these anti-MuSK antibodies, which is now widely accepted, remained controversial for a significant period following their initial description.

It has also become evident that some patients with MuSK-MG have an atypical clinical course and atypical findings on electromyography (EMG) studies. [1] Patients with MuSK-MG tend to have more prominent bulbar symptoms and more often have significant involvement of respiratory muscles and recurrent respiratory crises, compared to patients with AChR MG. Also in contrast to AChR-MG, a significant discrepancy is often found in patients with MuSK-MG between the clinical picture and EMG findings. Even during crisis and severe generalized weakness they do not show the same pattern in single-fiber EMG (SFEMG) that would have been seen with a similar clinical picture in a patient with classical AChR-MG. This can be partially explained by involvement of different muscle groups, but a significant difference in the EMG findings has also been found when patients with a similar degree of weakness in limb muscles were compared. [1, 2] However, the possibility that some MuSK-MG patients may have normal EMG studies, or, in other words, may present with no evidence of a neuromuscular transmission abnormality despite a myasthenic clinical picture, is still debated. This scenario has been discussed in a recent case report [32] and was also analyzed in one small group of patients whose antibodies were not detected by the usual assay but by a cell-based assay [3]. As the diagnosis of myasthenia in most centers relies on the detection of antibodies and/ or electrophysiological evidence of a neuromuscular transmission defect [4], it is quite likely that this group of patients, who have neither antibodies nor diagnostic EMG studies, has not been included in most laboratory studies performed to understand the pathophysiology of MuSK-MG. Thus, all animal studies of this illness demonstrate synaptic transmission abnormalities, lending further support to the notion that MuSK-MG always leads to abnormalities of synaptic transmission. Thus, only sporadic case reports and small series put this notion to question.

Despite the severity of the disease and non-satisfactory response to commonly used treatments and despite the difficulties in diagnosing MuSK-MG, there is surprisingly little clinical research aimed at finding better diagnostic approaches and treatment modalities, though in recent years there does seem to be a growing interest in this MG variant. [1, 5, 6] The single fiber EMG (SFEMG) test is seen by many neurologists as the diagnostic gold standard for MG, with a sensitivity approaching 100% [7], but is inherently incapable of detecting those (as-yet theoretical) abnormalities which affect muscle activity, resulting in a myasthenic clinical picture, but which have no effect on synaptic transmission, such as defects in those components of the neuromuscular junction which lie down-stream of the

AChR on the pathway from neuronal activation to muscular contraction. Thus, the SFEMG test may fail to detect an unknown number of MuSK-MG patients, who despite their fatigable muscle weakness will, on the basis of this widely employed test, be wrongly assumed to have a psychogenic or some ill-defined disease such as chronic fatigue syndrome [8]. This is concerning as such patients will be deprived of adequate treatment and even proper symptomatic and supportive care [9].

In this review we will present the case of one patient with an atypical clinical presentation and diagnostic studies [32]. Through this case we try to address the possible mechanisms involved in MuSK-MG when no synaptic transmission failure is found, and we suggest that this group of patients be studied more meticulously. We also stress the importance of gaining a better understanding of the underlying pathophysiology in providing better symptomatic and supportive care for patients who are refractory to immunomodulatory treatment, which is not a rare occurrence in this MG variant [10].

Case Presentation

Course of the Illness

A healthy 43-year-old hospital physician presented with a few weeks history of mild exertional dyspnea. Bronchial asthma was suspected and a salbutamol fixed dose inhaler led to some improvement. However, intermittent mild limb weakness, fatigue, significant weight loss and an episode of severe generalized weakness and dyspnea prompted further investigations. Her history was significant for a single brief episode of pyridostigmine-responsive ptosis and fatigable muscle weakness 15 years earlier. MG had then been excluded due to the normal ancillary tests and complete recovery. Current examination showed left eye ptosis, generalized limb weakness and speech dyspnea. MG was suspected and indeed, improvement was observed with pyridostigmine to the extent that she could resume her clinical duties for a short period, although she continued to suffer from relatively mild intermittent respiratory and swallowing difficulties. A sudden unprovoked episode of severe dyspnea with orthopnea and speech dyspnea at work a few months later caused ICU admission. Respiratory tests showed a maximum inspiratory pressure of -20 cmH_2O (normal <-60) and a maximum expiratory pressure of 50 cmH_2O (normal >100). Intravenous neostigmine led to a significant, transient improvement. Myasthenic crisis was diagnosed and plasmapheresis started. During these sessions episodes of near-paralysis appeared unexpectedly, managed with neostigmine and non-invasive ventilation (NIV). A severe, rare adverse reaction to citrate was suspected and could be partially controlled by calcium supplementation and decreasing citrate solution flow. Plasmapheresis achieved significant, but very short-lived, improvement. Further treatment trials with corticosteroids, azathioprine and IV immunoglobulins (IVIG) were ineffective or even led to worsening. Multiple serological and electrophysiological testing, including SFEMG of the orbicularis oculi and repetitive nerve stimulation (RNS) of the diaphragm were normal. Over the next 2 years, while treated with pyridostigmine and pacing her daily activities, she continued to have daily early morning awakenings with dyspnea, as well as episodes of more severe generalized weakness and respiratory difficulties. Her clinical course remained unusual with extreme and rapid changes in her muscle strength and functional ability. A discrepancy existed between the often normal standard neurological examinations and the degree of fatigability observed on more elaborate testing. A slow and gradual functional deterioration eventually prevented walking more than ~100 meters without significant dyspnea on most days, and a concomitant worsening of respiratory muscle forces and maximal voluntary ventilation was observed. A cardiopulmonary exercise stress test was significantly abnormal, with a VO2max of 30%-of-expected suggesting a possible metabolic abnormality. However, a deltoid muscle biopsy and an ischemic lactate stress test were normal. Unexpectedly, a tourniquet release following the lactate stress test led to transient severe generalized weakness and dyspnea.

Because of the unusual clinical course, negative ancillary tests and poor response to treatment, neurologists remained uncomfortable about the diagnosis of MG. A psychiatric etiology was considered but refuted by the consultant psychiatrist. Several episodes of acute respiratory failure necessitated intermittent NIV and referral to a large international neuromuscular center.

Extensive SFEMG, EMG and standard serological studies were again normal. However, a sleep study showed nocturnal CO2 retention. Direct measurement of diaphragmatic strength using magnetic nerve stimulation finally confirmed significant fatigable weakness (see appendix) .A novel cell-based assay revealed anti-MuSK antibodies. A 5-day plasmapheresis course soon enabled unassisted walking at a normal pace for a few hundred meters, the patient became free of respiratory support, and the quantitative MG score (QMG) improved from 20 to 12 However, as a regimen of escalating alternate day corticosteroids was instated, an unexpected gradual dose-dependent deterioration occurred to the extent that the patient became nearly bedridden, with recurrent episodic severe respiratory compromise mandating non-invasive ventilation (NIV) and deteriorating QMG to 22. This was initially ascribed to a transient paradoxical steroid-induced effect, but significant worsening, more pronounced on the days in which she took the steroids, continued. For the next few months (on 100mg prednisone q2d) she was incapacitated, unable to walk more than a few steps and suffering almost daily sudden episodes of severe generalized weakness and respiratory compromise requiring emergency respiratory support and neostigmine. Paradoxically, upon tapering down of the steroids she gradually improved and could partially resume hospital clinic work relying on frequent rest periods, intermittent respiratory support and a wheelchair for mobilization.

As steroid tapering continued, a trial of oral salbutamol (2 mg q8) led to gradual improvement in her endurance level and work capacity and to near-complete resolution of the more severe daily sudden episodes requiring emergent respiratory support, although she still required intermittent NIV. The addition of ephedrine (12mg q8), and substitution of salbutamol by a longer acting beta-agonist (Vospire 4mg q12) led to further improvement in her functional level, as did the addition of Mytelase (5 mg q8), an AChE inhibitor which was shown to be better tolerated in some patients with MuSK myasthenia.

Addition of Coenzyme Q10 and carnitine provided some improvement in endurance level. Episodes of more severe bulbar symptoms and respiratory crises were managed with minor changes in medications and supportive care, with a gradual recovery within a few weeks/months.

Details of Diagnostic Investigations and Possible Explanations

Serum antibodies (anti-AChR and anti-MuSK antibodies) were repeatedly negative. Anti-MuSK antibodies were eventually detected utilizing a cell-based assay (Figure 1). This assay was developed with the thought that better clustering of the AchR will enable detection of low affinity antibodies [11]. Indeed the detection of antibodies using this method was initially described in seronegative patients who had a typical and relatively mild classical AchR-MG. In the case described here the discrepancy between detection methods suggests either a different affinity of the antibodies to MuSK which can be overcome by antigen clustering on the cell membrane, but also the possibility of antibodies directed at an epitope which undergoes conformational changes when bound to other proteins, a phenomenon which has been described in other biological systems. [12] The latter explanation is more likely in view of the clinical picture.

EMG studies, consisting of RNS, SFEMG and needle EMG in numerous muscles, including the respiratory muscles, were performed numerous times, and were repeatedly negative. Thus, it is quite likely that the cause of the myasthenic clinical picture is not a result of neuromuscular junction (NMJ) transmission failure, but a down-stream excitation-contraction uncoupling. This finding suggests again that the anti-MuSK antibody in this case is directed at a different epitope which is not involved in NMJ assembly.

Effort-dependent respiratory tests ranged from near normal to significantly impaired, (see Figure 2), with an overall progressive pattern over the years of the illness.

Cardiorespiratory effort test showed a significant reduction in endurance level, with a VO2max of 30%. The overall pattern was consistent with findings in patients with mitochondrial myopathy.

Direct measurement of muscle force was performed using magnetic stimulation of the phrenic nerve, with measurements of pressure above and below the diaphragm as described [13]. This showed significant respiratory muscle weakness, with muscle fatigability, correlating with effort-dependent tests. (See appendix for detailed results.)

Noninvasive measurement of end-tidal CO_2 and oxygen saturation was done periodically. Oxygenation was well-preserved most of the time and never went below 90%. CO_2 levels were abnormally low at baseline and fluctuated in accordance with muscle strength (Figure 3).

A sleep study and noninvasive monitoring of O_2/CO_2 showed nocturnal hypoventilation with CO_2 retention, which significantly improved with non-invasive respiratory support.

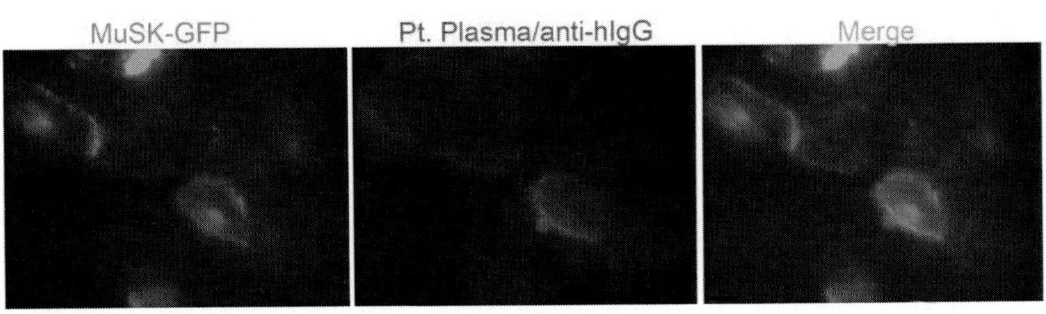

Figure 1. High-power fluorescence microscope images showing binding of antibodies in the patient's serum sample (red staining) to MuSK-EGFP (green staining) expressed on HEK cells.

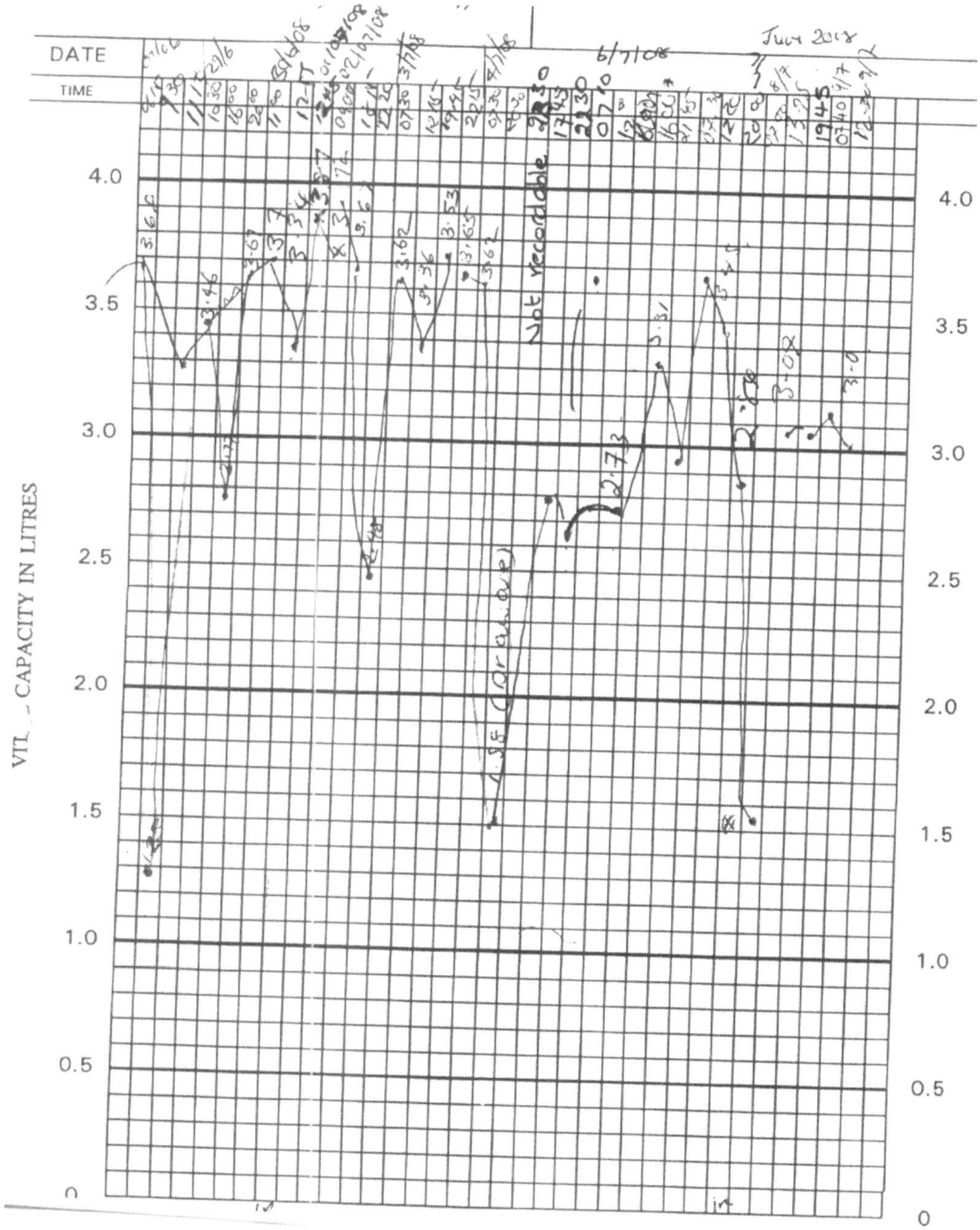

Figure 2. Respiratory tests invariably showed a fluctuative pattern: Measurement of vital capacity during hospitalization.

Details of Therapuetic Interventions

Pyridostigmine provided some symptomatic improvement but had an unpredictable effect and became less effective with time. The same dose could lead to improvement or worsening with frequent fasciculations. Anti-MuSK antibodies have a combined effect on acetylcholine levels. Both presynaptic, postsynaptic and a direct effect on acetylcholine esterase have been demonstrated. [14] This can lead to unpredictable levels of acetylcholine in the NMJ. Further more, a recent study showed a deleterious effect of pyridostigmine on AChR levels in patients with MuSK-MG [15]

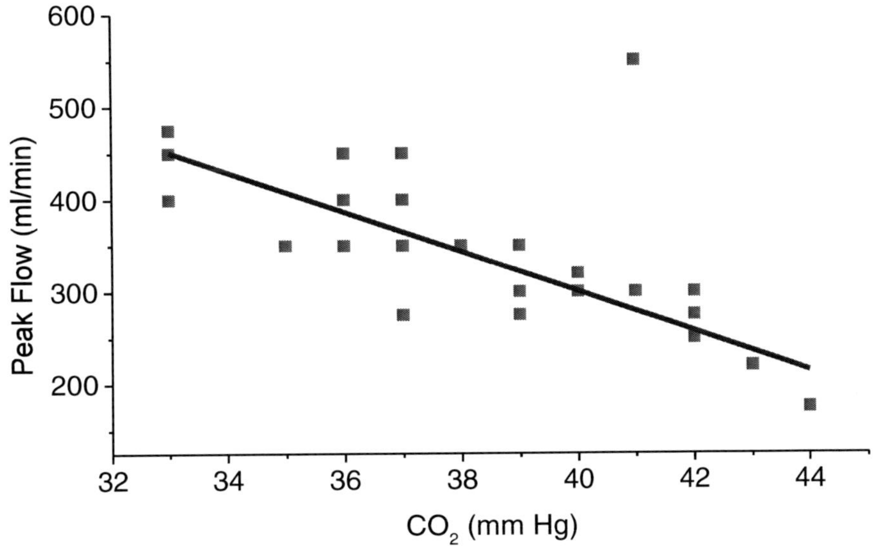

A

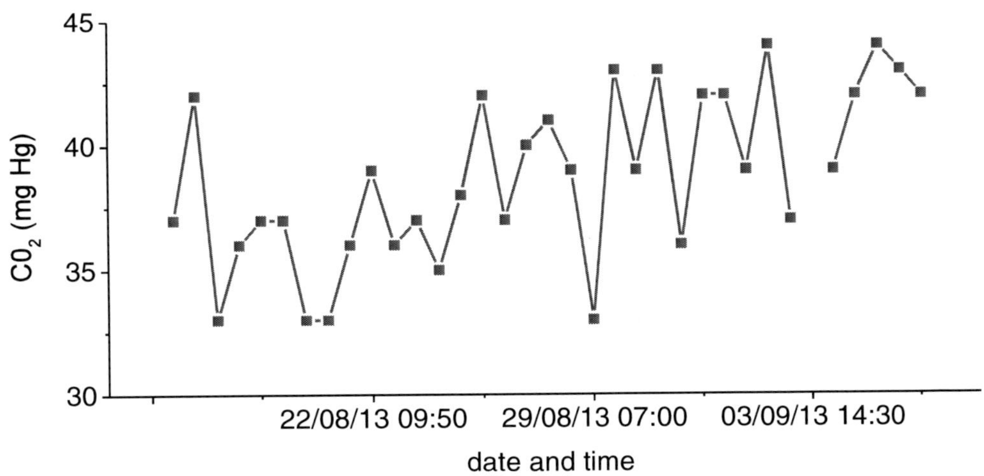

B

Figure 3. CO_2 levels measured using a hand-held capnometer. A. correlation of CO_2 levels and peak flow. B. typical two-week measurement of CO_2 levels during the day.

Plasmapheresis led to significant and rapid yet transient improvement. It also caused significant initial deterioration during the procedure itself. This has been described in MG patients and could be explained by increased sensitivity to calcium level shifts caused by citrate chelation. [16] Although calcium-induced calcium release is not a prominent mechanism in skeletal as opposed to cardiac muscle contraction, it has a significant role in muscle fatigability (see below).

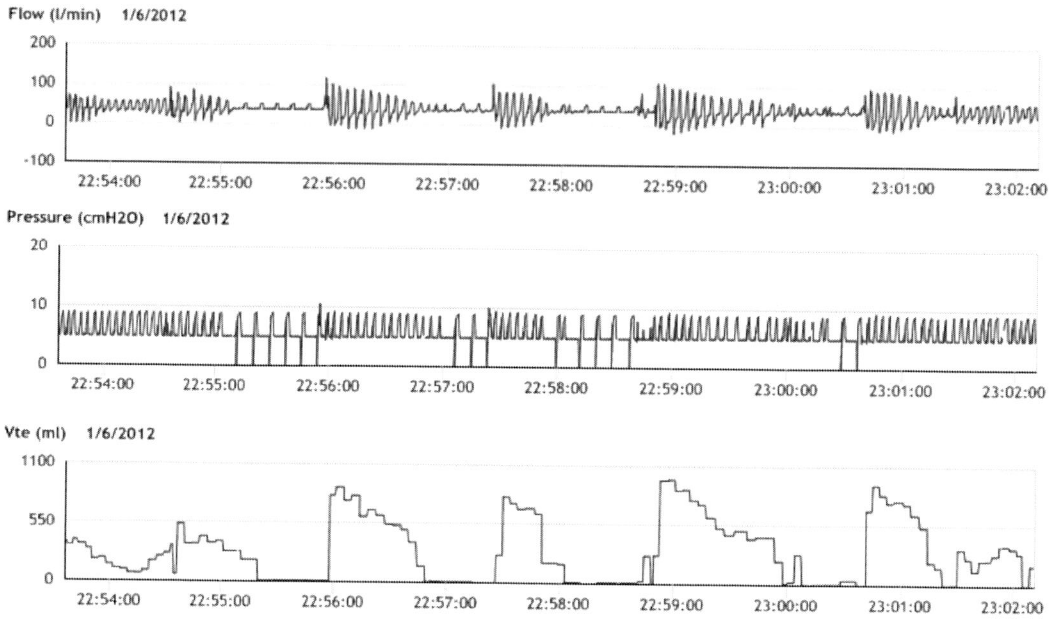

A

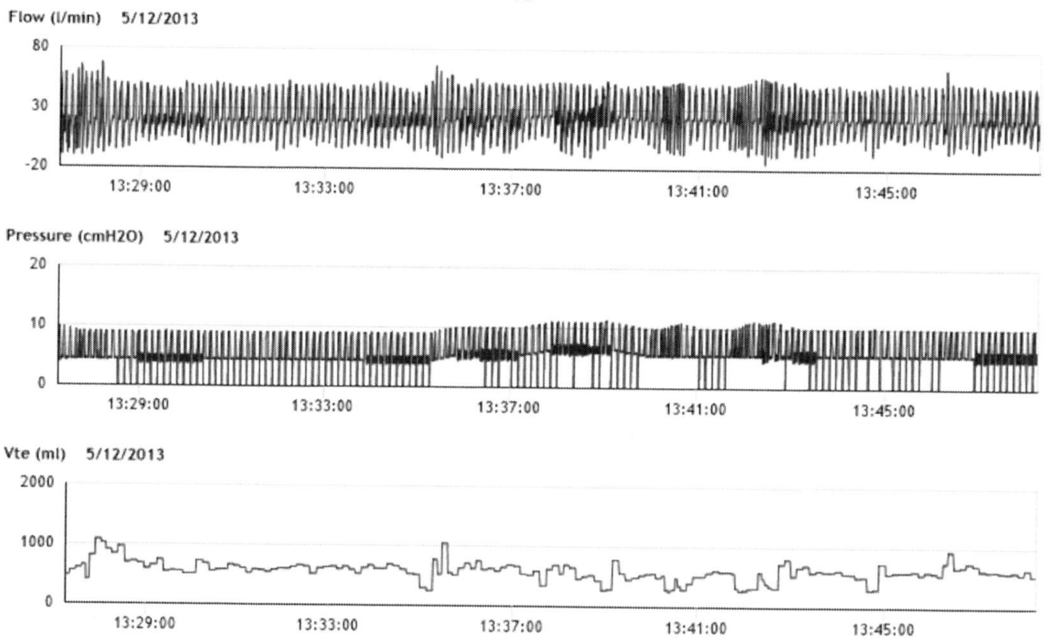

B

Figure 4. A. Tracing obtained from the respirator while using a fixed pressure mode. Note times in which flow and volume are inadequate. B. Tracing obtained from the respirator while using an AVASP-AE mode, in which both the inspiratory and expiratory pressure change according to the target volume. Note that volume is maintained at a near constant level while pressures range from EPAP-4-8 cm H_2O and IPAP-8-15 cm H_2O.

Steroids: Apart from their effect on the immune system, corticosteroids in pharmacological doses have numerous direct effects on skeletal muscle which can lead to acute or chronic changes [17]. Initial worsening of MG symptoms has been described [18]. Steroid myopathy in general is more common in MuSK MG [19].

Ventolin: Beta-2 adrenergic agonists such as salbutamol, apart from their well known bronchodilatory effect, have in a relatively high dose a direct effect on force generation by the diaphragm [20], and have been proposed in the management of a wide range of pathologies of skeletal muscles [21]. It has also been suggested that the action of salbutamol is coupled to the activation of the AChR complex and leads to the release of calcium from the SR. Indeed, salbutamol and other adrenergic agents have been shown to be beneficial in the treatment of certain types of congenital myasthenia [22].

Interestingly, even in patients with a good clinical response, no changes are documented in electrophysiological studies [23]. The remarkable symptomatic response achieved with those agents in our patient who had no NMJ transmission abnormalities, lends further support to a mode of action beyond the AChR complex, consistent with a possible effect on excitation-contraction coupling/calcium-related signaling [24–26], which was partially correctable by this treatment.

Mytelase: This longer acting acetylcholine esterase inhibitor was found to be better tolerated in some MG patients and specifically in MuSK [27].

NIV: Because of significant respiratory muscle involvement which ranged from relatively mild exertional dyspnea to near paralysis of the respiratory muscles, respiratory support was an essential component of treatment. The abnormally low CO_2 levels, combined with intermittent upper airway obstruction due to pharyngeal muscle weakness were not recognized initially. This led to settings which were not appropriate and caused numerous episodes of significant dyspnea and hypoventilation while using the respirator. Improvement was achieved by a more sensitive trigger, which allowed more patient triggered breathing and better synchrony, as well as volume-controlled respiration and dynamic changes of respiratory pressures. This was specifically achieved by Respironics Trilogy 100 and A-40 respirators. Because of the significant decrease in the work of breathing achieved, using the respirator for short periods led to significant recovery and improvement of respiratory force and much better sleep quality and day-time functioning. It also enabled treatment of crises in the ambulatory home setting during periods of worsening disease. (Figure 4).

Possible Mechanism

In order to understand the possible mechanism by which antibodies directed against MuSK may exert their effect; one has to understand the physiological basis of muscle contraction and metabolism as well as the possible role of MuSK in those processes. MuSK is a complex membrane protein with multiple domains. It has 3 extracellular Ig-like domains, a Frizzled domain (which binds the protein Wnt) and an intracellular catalytic domain. Although its role in embryonic development and NMJ formation is quite well understood, its role in mature muscle fibers is less well understood [5]. Yet, there is some evidence to suggest that MuSK may have an important role in excitation-contraction coupling or the translation of the electrical signal transmitted from the nerve ending to effective muscle contraction.

Muscle Contraction

Muscle contraction is a complex and well-orchestrated process, which involves many steps. The first step is transmission of the electrical signal from the nerve to the muscle. Once this occurs there is depolarization and entry of calcium into the cell, as well as release of calcium from intracellular stores.

Calcium and ATP are required for the proper function of the mechanochemical proteins actin and myosin. The energy-requiring sliding action of the actin and myosin leads to shortening of the muscle fiber, i.e., to muscle contraction. Not less important is the proper re-entry of calcium into the stores and the ensuing muscle relaxation, which allows the next muscle contraction to occur in a timely manner.

The force generated with each muscle contraction is regulated by calcium, cellular energy production and various extracellular mediators, such as epinephrine and cortisol. Muscle fibers are capable of rapid adaptation to changing requirements. They can rapidly go from a resting state of minimal energy production and utilization to massive energy expenditure.

Genetic or acquired abnormalities in any of the steps in this process can lead to muscle weakness, muscle fatigue, muscle necrosis, or any combination. Traditionally there is a division of those abnormalities to energy production defects, such as glycogen storage diseases or mitochondrial myopathies, calcium and other ion handling abnormalities such as periodic paralysis, neuromuscular transmission defects such as MG, and inflammatory changes such as polymyostis. In reality this is probably a relatively simplified approach as abnormalities in one step can many times lead to abnormalities in other steps and different pathophysiological processes can occur in the same disease. These include, for instance, the formation of reactive oxygen species (ROS), a byproduct of mitochondrial respiration that modulates cellular calcium, and abnormalities of glucose metabolism that can lead to abnormalities of oxidative phosphorylation and changes in ion channels and ion entry into the cell. Furthermore, many proteins have multiple functions, each of which may be affected by a disease process. Thus abnormalities in different domains of the same protein may lead to different cellular impairment and a different clinical presentation. Abnormalities of NMJ transmission and energy production can lead to a very similar clinical picture, as can be exemplified by the many clinical similarities between mitochondrial myopathies (MM) and myasthenia and the way one can mimic the other [28].

Calcium

Calcium is essential for muscle contraction. Upon depolarization of the muscle membrane, calcium is released from the sarcoplasmic reticulum (SR) [29, 30].

T-tubules are the major sites for the coupling of excitation and contraction, which is the process whereby the spreading depolarization is converted into force production by muscle fibers. The L-type calcium channels in T-tubules activate in response to electrical stimulation; their opening allows calcium to flow down its electrochemical gradient and into the cell.

Activation of the L-type channel also causes a mechanical interaction between it and calcium-release channels located on the adjacent sarcoplasmic reticulum membrane.

Although skeletal muscles are less dependent on extracellular calcium entry through the L-type channels than cardiac muscles, it should be realized that extracellular calcium levels and entry into the cell do modify muscle contraction [31]. This is not due to an effect on membrane de-polarization but rather on excitation-contraction coupling. When extracellular calcium is reduced, there is a decrease in the force of muscle contraction, despite normal excitation, upon repeat stimulation [31]. Under physiological conditions minor calcium level shifts are quite likely of little consequence as there are significant reserves for adequate muscle contraction, but they may have an effect under pathological conditions, when muscle reserves are limited [32].

Calcium release and calcium entry into the SR are highly regulated energy-requiring processes. Abnormalities in calcium release, calcium buffering and calcium re-entry can all lead to muscle fatigue and or impaired muscle relaxation [30].

Levels of intracellular calcium also effect levels of mitochondrial calcium, which in turn regulate ATP production by modulation of production of actetyl Co-A from pyruvate [29]. The T tubule system has sensors of ADP/ATP levels. Thus ATP production and calcium levels are tightly linked [30].

Calcium and Musk

MuSK does not directly bind calcium, but may indirectly be involved in its regulation, as both agrin-MuSK and wnt-MuSK interactions require calcium [33].

It is conceivable that calcium levels regulate MuSK function, although to the best of our knowledge this has not been studied. Calcium is important in wnt signaling, mostly in the non-canonical pathway that controls cell motility [34].

As cell motility and muscle contractions have many common features, it is possible that MuSK is involved in muscle contraction, through activation of actin. Activation of F-actin by MuSK has been demonstrated in neuronal cells.. Interestingly, although MuSK was initially thought to be confined to muscle fibers, it is now known that it is found in other motile cells such as sperm [35], highly suggesting that the role of MuSK in the adult (as opposed to the embryonic muscle) is not confined to the assembly of the NMJ.

Energy Production

ATP can be generated via glycolysis or oxidative phyosphrylation in which pyruvate or fatty acids can enter the mitochondrial tricarboxylic acid (TCA) cycle. There is a constant cross-talk between the mitochondria, the cytosol and the nucleus. Thus energy production in response to increasing cellular demands or quiescence is regulated by cytosolic and nuclear proteins as well as byproducts of those metabolic processes, such as lactate.

Impairment of mitochondrial function can therefore be a direct result of mitochondrial proteins, but also a result of abnormalities in various nuclear and cytosolic proteins. For instance: glycogen storage diseases, which should theoretically only effect glycolysis, have a significant effect on mitochondrial function as well [36].

MuSK and Energy Production

The role of MuSK in energy production and cell motility is not clear. Yet, as stated above it is unlikely that MuSK is only involved in NMJ assembly, as it is found in cells which lack such structures.

MuSK interacts with numerous proteins that have an effect on muscle metabolism and energy production, such as Wnt and LRP. MuSK has mostly been studied with regards to its role in NMJ assembly, but it is not likely that such a complex protein pathway will be abundant in mature cells only for this purpose. NMJ reassembly, maintenance and repair are tightly linked to cell activity; oxidative stress, etc. [37, 38], so it is more than conceivable that MuSK will be involved in those processes as well. This is indeed the case for LRP and Wnt.

MuSK-MG patients do not routinely undergo cardiorespiratory exercise testing, so there is very sparse data regarding such physiological abnormalities (see case description). Yet, in patients with MuSK-MG there is evidence for ultra-structural mitochondrial abnormalities suggesting that this may be more significant than previously appreciated.

The (Possible) Pathophisiology of Anti-musk Antibodies

It is now well recognized that anti-MuSK antibodies belong to the IgG4 subgroup and therefore exert their effect by modulating MuSK function and not by complement fixation and disruption [5]. There is a clear correlation between the level of anti-MuSK IgG4 and the clinical picture [39].

Variability in clinical presentation and electrophysiological findings suggests that anti-MuSK antibodies are not uniform and are quite likely directed at different epitopes of this large and complex protein. Indeed it was recently found that at least in some patients there are antibodies directed against the Frizzled domain. Those are not detected by the commonly used RIA, but only by using cell-based assays. [40].

Variability in laboratory studies [5] further supports the possibility of different antibodies targeting the same protein: some that have a more pronounced effect on the NMJ and others that may have a more pronounced effect on other cellular functions of MuSK.

Furthermore, both Wnt and LRP family proteins have a significant role in the regulation of metabolism/ mitochondrial function in numerous biological systems [34, 41, 42, 43]. MuSK and Wnt specifically have been shown to modulate F-actin in neuronal cells [44]. This makes it more than likely that disruption of their normal interaction with MuSK due toblocking antibodies will have an effect on muscle contraction and muscle energy production. Indeed, electron microscopy studies revealed prominent mitochondrial changes in muscle obtained from MuSK-MG patients as opposed to much more prominent NMJ changes in those obtained from AChR-MG patients. [45]. Unfortunately, metabolic studies are not routinely done in patients with myasthenia so there are no clinical correlates.

This variability of the antibodies could also explain why some patients with MuSK-MG have much less prominent or even null findings on SFEMG studies even in the face of severe disease, including myasthenic crisis. [1].

The fact that NMJ transmission abnormalities lead to abnormal muscle fatigability and weakness does not support the conclusion that muscle fatigability is invariably associated with such abnormalities. Abnormal muscle fatigability may be the result of defects in any step of the process leading to muscle contraction, including excitation-contraction coupling and energy production. [46, 47, 30]. Importantly the allegedly high sensitivity of SFEMG is seriously questioned in patients who are not anti-AChR positive. [48] One has to remember that the original clinical description of MG was that of muscle fatigability, which was also objectively demonstrated by Jolly [49].

Emerging knowledge regarding MuSK highly suggests that it has a pivotal role in effective muscle contraction by orchestrating EP signaling, EM coupling and energy metabolism via its various ligands.

Therefore abnormalities of MuSK function can lead to muscle fatigue in more than one way. Quite likely, in some patients more than one mechanism is at play, whereas in others a certain mechanism is more prominent. This will in turn dictate the severity of the disease and the type of muscles involved. It may also lead to a very complex clinical picture.

For instance, a combination of decreased electro-mechanical coupling with decreased energy production, may lead to a very confusing, severe and seemingly paradoxical clinical picture in which respiratory muscle weakness and fatigability leading to hypoventilation will not be accompanied by significant CO_2 retention or hypoxemia. In fact, CO2 levels may be decreased instead of increased despite normal or even hypoventilation due to significant decrease in CO_2 production by the muscles because of abnormalities in mitochondrial energy production, accompanied by a similar decrease in O_2 consumption, as is seen in mitochondrial myopathies [50–53]. Relatively mild CO_2 retention and hypoxemia will only occur once respiratory muscle dysfunction is severe enough to hamper even the decreased CO_2 production and O_2 consumption. Periodic breathing during sleep and exertion may be the result of this interplay between decreased CO2 production and alternating severity of respiratory muscle dysfunction.

This putative mechanism may also have therapeutic implications as it will dictate respiratory settings in patients requiring NIV (see case description), and possibly the use of food supplements known to improve mitochondrial energy production in other diseases.

Management

The management consists of the combination of pharmacological treatment, supportive care and life-style changes as required.

The current pharmacological management approach has recently been reviewed [38]. In general, patients with MuSK-MG tend to have a more severe illness, recurrent crises and poor response to treatment as in the case described. The treatment options for patients with refractory disease are limited and consist of experimental treatment, such as Rituximab which showed promising results in small case series and sporadic cases, but for which there is lack of knowledge regarding long term effects and risks.

Symptomatic treatment can also pose a difficulty as many patients do not benefit from treatment with pyridostigmine. Other acetylcholine esterase inhibitors such as mytelase may be better tolerated, as well as adrenergic agents such as salbutamol.

Noninvasive ventilation is a well-established therapy in patient with chronic respiratory failure due to different neuromuscular pathologies and severe chest wall abnormalities [54, 55]. Nocturnal respiratory failure in patients with neuromuscular disorders including MG might be treated by NIV [56] Some evidence about the efficacy of NIV in acute worsening of patients with mysthenia gravis is present in the literature [57, 58] . The importance of different lung function test and blood gases parameters was demonstrated, predicting either the timing to start mechanical ventilation or prognosis of survival in patients admitted to the intensive care unit due to acute neuromuscular respiratory failure [59] and specifically in myasthenia [60].This scanty data provides the indications and timing of supportive ventilation both for MG crisis and chronic respiratory failure secondary to this neuromuscular disease.

Adequate nutrition is of paramount importance in a disease with impaired muscle function. Yet, many patients with MuSK-MG suffer from varying levels of bulbar symptoms which may significantly affect their oral intake at times. Ideally patients should be followed by a speech therapist and dietician who can periodically adjust the nutritional mode and intake according to the patient's condition. Not less important is adjustment of the home and work place environment by an occupational therapist and physiotherapist as required, using tools and aids which allow maximal function even during times of more significant weakness and also decrease the strain on the muscles to avoid reaching a high level of fatigue.

Learning to utilize the limited energy in the most efficient way can significantly aid in leading a productive life. Patients should be taught how to recognize early signs of weakness and promptly rest. Patients should be encouraged to do as much as they can without exceeding their limits. This is not trivial and requires support and education.

The changing and unpredictable nature of the illness combined with the at many times disappointing results of treatment, puts an inevitable strain on the physician-patient relationship. This should be honestly addressed. A warm and supportive environment, based on mutual trust and respect, and a multidisciplinary approach which also involves the patient in decision making are very important in this complex disease with overall limited treatment options.

Conclusion

Patients with MuSK-MG pose a significant diagnostic and management problem, as has also been demonstrated by the case described. This is mostly because although many of the clinical features of their illness highly resemble standard MG, there are numerous clinical features and findings that do not fit.

Before the detection of anti-MuSK antibodies this illness with many times normal diagnostic tests was not seen as a "real" disease and even patients with severe respiratory symptoms were given various psychiatric diagnoses and received fragmented and inadequate treatment. (9). This, to some extent, was also the case for the patient described, who being a physician herself was better able to orchestrate her own care. Even putting MuSK-MG patients in the procrustean bed of AChR-aMG may not be beneficial, as this disease is distinct in its underlying pathophysiology and many of the treatments are ineffective and possibly harmful [61].

Even now, more than a decade later, the knowledge and understanding of this illness is still lacking due to several factors. Firstly, it is relatively rare. Secondly, it is still disputed by many neurologists that MG can be diagnosed in the face of normal EMG studies or that myasthenia does not equate with NMJ transmission abnormalities, so possibly the reason for the low prevalence is misdiagnosis. Thirdly, the unusual features of this illness are many times attributed to emotional problems [62] instead of realizing the complexity of its pathophysiology and trying to gain a better understanding of the underlying pathophysiology. Finally, the vast majority of the biological and clinical data regarding MuSK-MG is derived from patients who have electrophysiological abnormalities, thus missing other potential mechanisms not related to NMJ transmission effects, whose identification may possibly lead to better management approaches for the entire patient population.

Despite the severity of this illness, there are no clinical trials directed at MuSK-MG patients. In fact most MG clinical trials actually exclude them. Many patients do not even receive adequate symptomatic and supportive care directed at improving their functional level, even if not altering the course of the disease. There are no studies looking at the use of NIV in MuSK-MG patients with respiratory muscle involvement, for instance.

A better understanding of the pathophysiology of MuSK MG can lead not only to better treatment of this illness, but also to better understanding of the physiology of muscle function in health and disease.

Currently available tools which assess excitation-contraction coupling [26], endurance [53], muscle force and fatigability [63] are not widely used or standardized for this patient population. Such improvement in objective assessment tools will allow better diagnosis and better follow up of response to treatment.

Further studies looking at the entire MuSK-MG patient population, looking specifically for those with no evidence for NMJ transmission defects with meticulous clinical and pathophysiological correlations, are highly required and will likely lead to gaining better knowledge of the true prevalence of MuSK-MG, better management approaches and better understanding of the underlying pathophysiology.

Acknowledgment

The valuable contributions of Prof. A. Vincent in the cell-based assays; of Prof. A. Simonds in the magnetic stimulation tests; and of Prof. G. Haran and Arnon Haran in the critical reading of this manuscript are gratefully acknowledged.

Conflicts of Interest

None to declare.

Appendix

Results of Effort dependent respiratory tests and direct measurement of diaphragmatic force and fatigability.

Problems:			
Reason for referral Suspected myasthenia gravis possible affecting respiratory muscles On nocturnal non-invasive ventilation			
GLOBAL MUSCLE STRENGTH (cmH2O)		Predicted	Observed
	INSPIRATORY		
	Sniff Oesophageal Pressure (Poes)	>60	24
	Sniff Nasal Pressure (SNIP)	>70 (M) >60 (F)	20
	EXPIRATORY		
	Cough Gastric Pressure (Pgas)	>120	77
DIAPHRAGM STRENGTH (cmH_2O)		Predicted	Observed
	Sniff Transdiaphragmatic Pressure (Sniff Pdi)	>80	20
	Bilateral Anterior Stimulation (TwPdi)	>20	Not done
	Left Unilateral Stimulation (TwPdi)	>8	4.3
	Right Unilateral Stimulation (TwPdi)	>7	3.5
DYNAMIC COMPLIANCE ($L.cmH2O^{-1}$)		0.1-0.35	Not done
COMMENTS On repetitive magnetic phrenic nerve stimulation over 40 seconds, left TwPdi dropped from 4.3 to 2.8, right TwPdi went from 3.5 to 3.			

References

[1] Stickler, D. E., Massey, J. M. & Sanders, D. B. MuSK-antibody positive myasthenia gravis: clinical and electrodiagnostic patterns. *Clinical neurophysiology: official journal of the International Federation of Clinical Neurophysiology* 116, 2065–8 (2005).

[2] Farrugia, M. E., Kennett, R. P., Newsom-Davis, J., Hilton-Jones, D. & Vincent, A. Single-fiber electromyography in limb and facial muscles in muscle-specific kinase antibody and acetylcholine receptor antibody myasthenia gravis. *Muscle & nerve* 33, 568–70 (2006).

[3] Farrugia, M. E., Leite, I., Petty, R., Overell, J. A., Mallik, A., and Vincent, A., in *XIIth International Congress on Neuromuscolar Diseases* (Napoli, 2010).

[4] Argov, Z. Current approach to seronegative myasthenia. *Journal of neurology* 258, 14–8 (2011).

[5] Koneczny, I., Cossins, J. & Vincent, A. The role of muscle-specific tyrosine kinase (MuSK) and mystery of MuSK myasthenia gravis. *Journal of anatomy* (2013).

[6] Chroni, E. & Punga, A. R. Neurophysiological characteristics of MuSK antibody positive Myasthenia Gravis mice: focal denervation and hypersensitivity to acetylcholinesterase inhibitors. *Journal of the neurological sciences* 316, 150–7 (2012).

[7] Juel, V. C. & Massey, J. M. Myasthenia gravis. *Orphanet journal of rare diseases* 2, 44 (2007).

[8] Wessely, S. & Powell, R. Fatigue syndromes: a comparison of chronic "postviral" fatigue with neuromuscular and affective disorders. *Journal of neurology, neurosurgery, and psychiatry* 52, 940–8 (1989).

[9] Chloe G, K. Atkins., *My Imaginary illness: a journey into uncertainty and prejudice in medical diagnosis.* (Cornell university press, Ithaca and London, 2010).

[10] Suh, J., Goldstein, J. M. & Nowak, R. J. Clinical characteristics of refractory myasthenia gravis patients. Yale J Biol Med. 86, 255–260 (2013).

[11] Leite, M. I. et al. IgG1 antibodies to acetylcholine receptors in "seronegative" myasthenia gravis. *Brain: a journal of neurology* 131, 1940–52 (2008).

[12] Casolini, F. et al. Antibody response to fibronectin-binding adhesin FnbpA in patients with Staphylococcus aureus infections. *Infection and immunity* 66, 5433–42 (1998).

[13] Luo, Y. M. et al. Reproducibility of twitch and sniff transdiaphragmatic pressures. *Respiratory physiology & neurobiology* 132, 301–6 (2002).

[14] Niks, E. H. et al. Pre- and postsynaptic neuromuscular junction abnormalities in musk myasthenia. *Muscle & nerve* 42, 283–8 (2010).

[15] Morsch, M., Reddel, S. W., Ghazanfari, N., Toyka, K. V & Phillips, W. D. Pyridostigmine but not 3,4-diaminopyridine exacerbates ACh receptor loss and myasthenia induced in mice by muscle-specific kinase autoantibody. *The Journal of physiology* 591, 2747–62 (2013).

[16] Wirguin, I., Brenner, T., Shinar, E. & Argov, Z. Citrate-induced impairment of neuromuscular transmission in human and experimental autoimmune myasthenia gravis. *Annals of neurology* 27, 328–30 (1990).

[17] Kumar, S. Steroid-induced myopathy following a single oral dose of prednisolone. *Neurology India* 51, 554–6 (2003).

[18] Bae, J. S., Go, S. M. & Kim, B. J. Clinical predictors of steroid-induced exacerbation in myasthenia gravis. *Journal of clinical neuroscience: official journal of the Neurosurgical Society of Australasia* 13, 1006–10 (2006).

[19] Evoli, A. et al. Response to therapy in myasthenia gravis with anti-MuSK antibodies. *Annals of the New York Academy of Sciences* 1132, 76–83 (2008).

[20] Laghi, F., Tobin, M. J. & Hatipo, G. Does inhaled albuterol improve contractility in Patients with Chronic Obstructive Pulmonary Disease? American Journal of Respiratory and Critical Care Medicine, Vol. 160, No. 6 (1999), pp. 1916-1921.

[21] Lynch, G. S. & Ryall, J. G. Role of β-Adrenoceptor Signaling in Skeletal Muscle: Implications for Muscle Wasting and Disease. *Physiological Reviews* 729–767 (2008). .

[22] Liewluck, T., Selcen, D. & Engel, A. G. Beneficial effects of albuterol in congenital endplate acetylcholinesterase deficiency and Dok-7 myasthenia. *Muscle & nerve* 44, 789–94 (2011).

[23] Lashley, D., Palace, J., Jayawant, S., Robb, S. & Beeson, D. Ephedrine treatment in congenital myasthenic syndrome due to mutations in DOK7. *Neurology* 74, 1517–23 (2010).

[24] Imai, T. et al. Contribution of anti-ryanodine receptor antibody to impairment of excitation-contraction coupling in myasthenia gravis. *Clinical neurophysiology: official journal of the International Federation of Clinical Neurophysiology* 123, 1242–7 (2012).

[25] Nakata, M. et al. Is excitation-contraction coupling impaired in myasthenia gravis? *Clinical neurophysiology: official journal of the International Federation of Clinical Neurophysiology* 118, 1144–8 (2007).

[26] Tsuda, E. et al. Correlation of bite force with excitation-contraction coupling time of the masseter in myasthenia gravis. *Clinical neurophysiology: official journal of the International Federation of Clinical Neurophysiology* 121, 1051–8 (2010).

[27] Farrugia, M. E., Melms, A. & Vincent, A. Myasthenia gravis with MuSK antibodies. Practical neurology. 356–359 (2005).

[28] Whittaker, R. G., Schaefer, A. M., Taylor, R. W. & Turnbull, D. M. Differential diagnosis in ptosis and ophthalmoplegia: mitochondrial disease or myasthenia? *Journal of neurology* 254, 1138–9 (2007).

[29] Berchtold, M. W., Brinkmeier, H. & Müntener, M. Calcium ion in skeletal muscle: its crucial role for muscle function, plasticity, and disease. *Physiological reviews* 80, 1215–65 (2000).

[30] Allen, D. G., Lamb, G. D. & Westerblad, H. Skeletal Muscle Fatigue: Cellular Mechanisms. *Physiological Reviews* 287–332 (2008)..

[31] Dulhunty, B. Y. A. F. & Gage, P. W. Effects of Extracellular Calcium Concentration Skeletal Muscle. 63–80 (1988).

[32] Haran, M. et al. Can a rare form of myasthenia gravis shed additional light on disease mechanisms? *Clinical neurology and neurosurgery* 1–5 (2012).

[33] Wu, H., Xiong, W. C. & Mei, L. To build a synapse: signaling pathways in neuromuscular junction assembly. *Development (Cambridge, England)* 137, 1017–33 (2010).

[34] Kohn, A. D. & Moon, R. T. Wnt and calcium signaling: beta-catenin-independent pathways. *Cell calcium* 38, 439–46 (2005).

[35] Kumar, P., Ferns, M. J. & Meizel, S. Identification of agrinSN isoform and muscle-specific receptor tyrosine kinase (MuSK) [corrected] in sperm. *Biochemical and biophysical research communications* 342, 522–8 (2006).

[36] Stefano, N. D. E., Argov, Z. & Matthews, P. M. Impairment of Muscle Mitochondrial Oxidative Metabolism In Mcardle ' S Disease. *Muscle Nerve.* 19, 764–769 (1996).

[37] Karalaki, M., Fili, S., Philippou, A. & Koutsilieris, M. Muscle regeneration: cellular and molecular events. *In vivo (Athens, Greece)* 23, 779–96 (2009).

[38] Evoli, A., Alboini, P. E., Bisonni, A., Mastrorosa, A. & Bartocccioni, E. Management challenges in muscle-specific tyrosine kinase myasthenia gravis. *Annals of the New York Academy of Sciences* 1274, 86–91 (2012).

[39] Niks, E. H. et al. Clinical fluctuations in MuSK myasthenia gravis are related to antigen-specific IgG4 instead of IgG1. *Journal of neuroimmunology* 195, 151–6 (2008).

[40] Takamori, M., Nakamura, T. & Motomura, M. Antibodies against Wnt receptor of muscle-specific tyrosine kinase in myasthenia gravis. *Journal of neuroimmunology* 254, 183–6 (2013).

[41] Rampazzo, E. et al. Wnt activation promotes neuronal differentiation of Glioblastoma. *Cell death & disease* 4, e500 (2013).

[42] Liu, W. et al. Low density lipoprotein (LDL) receptor-related protein 6 (LRP6) regulates body fat and glucose homeostasis by modulating nutrient sensing pathways and mitochondrial energy expenditure. *The Journal of biological chemistry* 287, 7213–23 (2012).

[43] Stiegler, A. L., Burden, S. J. & Hubbard, S. R. Crystal structure of the frizzled-like cysteine-rich domain of the receptor tyrosine kinase MuSK. *Journal of molecular biology* 393, 1–9 (2009).

[44] Banerjee, S. et al. A novel role for MuSK and non-canonical Wnt signaling during segmental neural crest cell migration. *Development (Cambridge, England)* 138, 3287–96 (2011).

[45] Cenacchi, G. et al. Comparison of muscle ultrastructure in myasthenia gravis with anti-MuSK and anti-AChR antibodies. *Journal of neurology* 258, 746–52 (2011).

[46] Verburg, E., Dutka, T. L. & Lamb, G. D. Long-lasting muscle fatigue: partial disruption of excitation-contraction coupling by elevated cytosolic Ca^{2+} concentration during contractions. *American journal of physiology. Cell physiology* 290, C1199–208 (2006).

[47] Chetta, A. & Aiello, M. Assessment of respiratory muscle fatigue in patients with neuromuscular diseases: a non-invasive approach. *Respiration; international review of thoracic diseases* 73, 412–3 (2006).

[48] Haran, M. In response to "current approach to seronegative myasthenia" by Z. Argov. *Journal of neurology* 258, 164–5 (2011).

[49] Hughes, T. The early history of myasthenia gravis. *Neuromuscular disorders: NMD* 15, 878–86 (2005).

[50] Heinicke, K. et al. Exertional dyspnea in mitochondrial myopathy: clinical features and physiological mechanisms. *Am J Physiol Regul Integr Comp Physiol*. 301 (2011).

[51] Je, C. Mitochondrial Disorders and Exertional Intolerance: Controversy Continues. *American Journal of Respiratory and Critical Care Medicine* 2–4 (1997).

[52] Punga, A. R., Ahlqvist, K., Bartoccioni, E., Scuderi, F. & Marino, M. Neurophysiological and mitochondrial abnormalities in MuSK antibody seropositive myasthenia gravis compared to other immunological subtypes. *Clinical Neurophysiology* 117, 1434–1443 (2006).

[53] Taivassalo, T. et al. The spectrum of exercise tolerance in mitochondrial myopathies: a study of 40 patients. *Brain* 126 (Pt 2):413-23 (2003).

[54] Simonds, A. K. Recent advances in respiratory care for neuromuscular disease. *Chest* 130, 1879–86 (2006).

[55] Shneerson, J. M. & Simonds, a. K. Noninvasive ventilation for chest wall and neuromuscular disorders. *European Respiratory Journal* 20, 480–487 (2002).

[56] Barthlen GM, Nocturnal respiratory failure as an indication of noninvasive ventilation in the patient with neuromuscular disease. *Respiration* 64 Suppl 1:35-8 (1997).

[57] Seneviratne, J., Mandrekar, J., Wijdicks, E. F. M. & Rabinstein, A. a. Noninvasive ventilation in myasthenic crisis. *Archives of neurology* 65, 54–8 (2008).

[58] Rabinstein, A. & Wijdicks, E. F. M. BiPAP in acute respiratory failure due to myasthenic crisis may prevent intubation. *Neurology* 59, 1647–9 (2002).

[59] Cabrera Serrano, M. & Rabinstein, a a. Usefulness of pulmonary function tests and blood gases in acute neuromuscular respiratory failure. *European journal of neurology: the official journal of the European Federation of Neurological Societies* 19, 452–6 (2012).

[60] Wu, J.-Y. et al. The role of non-invasive ventilation and factors predicting extubation outcome in myasthenic crisis. *Neurocritical care* 10, 35–42 (2009).

[61] Vincent, A., Bowen, J., Newsom-davis, J. & Mcconville, J. Seronegative generalised myasthenia gravis: clinical features , antibodies , and their targets Seronegative myasthenia gravis. *Lancet Neurology* 2, 99–106 (2003).

[62] Paul, R. H., Cohen, R. a, Goldstein, J. M. & Gilchrist, J. M. Severity of mood, self-evaluative, and vegetative symptoms of depression in myasthenia gravis. *The Journal of neuropsychiatry and clinical neurosciences* 12, 499–501 (2000).

[63] Schols, A. M. W. J., Moxham, J. & Polkey, M. I. A novel technique for nonvolitional assessment of quadriceps muscle endurance in humans. *Journal of Applied Physiology* 739–746 (2010).

In: Rare Diseases
Editors: Giorgio Di Giovanni and Pietro Marcoz

ISBN: 978-1-62948-525-6

Chapter IV

Main Forms and Neurological Complications of Histiocytosis

Eva Viragh[1], Csaba B. Nagy[2], Zoltan Locsei[1], Csaba Toth[3], Ferenc Garzuly[3] and Bernadette Kalman[4,*]

[1]Department of Medicine, Markusovszky University Hospital, Szombathely, Hungary
[2]Department of Radiology, Markusovszky University Hospital, Szombathely, Hungary
[3]Department of Pathology, Markusovszky University Hospital, Szombathely, Hungary
[4]Center for Research and Education, Markusovszky University Hospital, Szombathely, Hungary

Abstract

Histiocytosis represents a group of rare diseases presenting with different demographic, clinical, imaging, histological and molecular characteristics. The primary molecular pathology arises in and causes proliferation of tissue macrophages or histiocytes, elements of the lymphoreticular system.

The three most commonly encountered forms, Langerhans cell histiocytosis (LCH), Erdheim-Chester Disease (ECD) and Rosai-Dorfman disease (RDD), typically affect pediatric, adult, and pediatric - young adult age groups, respectively.

The range and severity of organ involvements span from a single organ (e.g., cutis) disease with good prognosis to multiple, high-risk organ (e.g., heart, lung, brain, bone marrow) involvements with increased morbidity and mortality.

When clinical and paraclinical data raise the suspicion for the entity, histological and immunohistochemical examination of lesions can verify the diagnosis and the actual subtype of histiocytosis. Involvement of the central nervous system (CNS) is common in each form, and is associated with significant diagnostic and treatment challenges.

While evidence-based information from placebo-controlled, randomized and double-blind trials is as yet unavailable, empirical data provide useful guidance for choosing effective treatment modalities in each of these conditions.

* Markusovszky Teaching Hospital of the University of Pecs, Markusovszky Street 5. 9700. Szombathely, Hungary.

Recent studies also reveal molecular substrates of transformation from tissue residential to pathological histiocytes, highlight the importance of acquired somatic mutations in the pathogenesis and identify potential new targets for therapy.

Keywords: Histiocytosis, central nervous system, somatic mutation, pathogenesis, treatment

Introduction

Histiocytosis represents a group of rare disorders characterized by cell proliferation in the mononuclear phagocytic lineage. The subgroup of bone marrow – derived monocytes that reaches various tissues and organs by blood circulation, is called histiocytes (related terms include tissue macrophages and dendritic cells) (Arico et al., 2003, Badalian-Very et al., 2012, Haroche et al., 2012). These cells are part of the mononuclear phagocytic (or lymphoreticular) system, and subject of molecular changes resulting in abnormal proliferation and histiocytosis (see details below).

The spectrum of clinical presentations is broad and ranges from benign, single system disease to life-threatening multiorgan involvement. In about half of the cases, histiocytosis also presents with central nervous system (CNS) involvements. Here we summarize main characteristics of Langerhans cell histiocytosis (LCH), Erdheim-Chester Disease (ECD), and Rosai-Dorfman disease (RDD), the most recognized subgroups of histiocytosis, and highlight neurological complications associated with these conditions (Arico et al., 2003, Badalian-Very et al., 2012, Postini et al., 2012, Haroche et al., 2012, Cavalli et al., 2013, Wilejto and Alba, 2012, Rosai and Dorfman, 1969). The three subentities are distinguished based on age of onset, distribution of pathology, clinical presentation, and immunohistochemical characteristics of the lesions (Table 1).

Recent advances in molecular genetics reveal that histiocytosis may be caused by somatic mutations in the mononuclear phagocytic lineage or its precursors, placing these conditions in close proximity with hematological malignancies. The benign self-limited variants at the one end and occasional coexistence of lympho- / hematologic disorders with histiocytosis at the other end of the clinical spectrum not only indicate the variability of phenotypes, but also suggest a temporal evolution and increasing complexity of underlying somatic genetic alterations (Arico et al., 2003, Badalian-Very et al., 2012, Postini et al., 2012, Haroche et al., 2012, Cavalli et al., 2013, Wilejto and Alba, 2012, Rosai and Dorfman, 1969). Because of the rarity of histiocytosis, both establishing the diagnosis and choosing the right disease modifying treatment can be challenging. However, in case of clinical suspicion, histological and immunohistochemical characterizations of a lesion will allow verification of the diagnosis and the actual histiocytosis subtype (Haroche et al., 2012). Molecular genetic testing of granulomas for certain recurrent somatic mutations may also be feasible at most centers with onco-hematological laboratory capabilities, which may reveal potential targets for newer therapeutic interventions to be considered along with the more traditional immune and chemotherapeutic modalities (Haroche et al., 2013, Landi et al., 2013).

This overview of current data on LCH, ECD and RDD aims to assist clinical management of these rare conditions and to highlight recent research accomplishments that facilitate better understanding of disease pathogenesis as well as support new treatment strategies.

Table 1.

	Langerhans cell histiocytosis	Erdheim-Chester disease	Rosai-Dorfman disease
Typical age of onset	Childhood	Adulthood	Childhood and young adulthood
Clinical manifestation, organs involvement	Bones (demarcated lytic lesion), skin, periodontal region, lung, liver, spleen, bone marrow, lymphoid organs infiltration Worse prognosis with younger age of onset and multiple, high risk organ involvement	Long bones (bilateral-symmetric cortical osteosclerosis), skin, kidney, lung, pericardium, wall of the heart, aorta and other arteries, retroperitoneum Worse prognosis with extensive pathology and high risk organ involvement	Bilateral painless massive cervical lymphadenopathy, skin, nasal cavity, paranasal sinuses, eyelids, orbit, bone, salivary gland Often spontaneous remission and benign prognosis; more severe presentation is also possible
CNS lesions	24-55% of cases: 1) granulomatous lesions in the cerebral connective tissue with or without parenchymal infiltration: meninges, choroid plexus, pituitary gland (diabetes insipidus, hormone deficiencies) and other focal parenchymal lesions 2) neurodegenerative lesions with neuronal loss, demyelination and gliosis: cerebellum, dentate nuclei, brain stem, basal ganglia (paraneoplastic?)	15-25% of cases: corticospinal and spinothalamic tracts, dorsal columns, cerebellar, meningeal, retroorbital, pituitary gland, cranial nerve involvements Presentation may be neuronal focal, cognitive, convulsive or psychiatric; may mimic MS	<5% of cases: leptomeninges (dural mass may be mimicking meningioma), brain (cerebral mass may be mimicking glioma), spinal cord
Immune phenotype	IHC: CD1a+, S100+, langerin (CD207)+ EM: Birbeck granules	IHC: CD1a-, CD68+, S100 +/-	IHC: CD1a-, CD68+, S100+ Emperipolesis present
Molecular characteristics	Clonal expansion of monocytoid cells / histiocytes with somatic mutations (e.g., ^{V600E}B-RAF)	Clonal origin is unclear; somatic (e.g., ^{V600E}B-RAF) mutations, rearrangements may be present	Less well characterized Etiology unclear Abnormal Fas/FasL signaling
Treatment, therapy	Cutaneous lesions: may spontaneously resolve; topical steroid, thalidomide, methotrexate, psoralen, long-wave UV radiation Organ involvement: combined and aggressive chemotherapy (cytarabine, cladribine), clofarabine, vemurafenib (B-RAF inhibitor) Pituitary involvement: -hormonal replacement	High dose IFN-α, pegylated IFN-α, steroid, cladribine, IL-1 receptor antagonist, autologous hemopoietic cell transplantation, hormonal replacement, vemurafenib (B-RAF inhibitor)	Spontaneous remission; surgical resection, steroid, irradiation, chemotherapy

1. Langerhans Cell Histiocytosis (LCH)

This disease subtype was described in 1953 as histiocytosis X, and sorted into four subgroups: 1) a self-limiting congenital form or Hashimoto-Pritzker disease; 2) a multifocal form with diabetes insipidus, exophthalmos and bone involvement or Hand-Schüller-Christian disease; 3) an intertriginous form or Letterer-Siwe disease and 4) a unifocal form of eosinophilic granuloma (Lichtenstein et al., 1953). Histiocytosis X was then re-classified by the Histiocyte Society as LCH, a single entity with a broad spectrum of clinical presentations (Writing Group of the Histiocyte Society, 1987).

The incidence of LCH is 4-8 cases / 1 million children / year (Stalemark et al., 2008, Oliveira et al., 2012). The incidence in adults is 1-2 cases / 1 million / year, with a mean age of 35 ± 14 years, and is more prevalent in males (Arico et al., 2003, Lajolo et al., 2012).

The highly variable presentation and prognosis depend on the age of onset, the distribution of pathology to a single or multiple organs (skin, bone, periodontal or gum regions, lung, liver, spleen, lymphoid organs, bone marrow, brain, pituitary gland, etc..), and the aggressiveness of the progression (Oliveira et al., 2012, Postini et al. 2012, Gupta and Bansal, 2012). Postini et al. (2012) reviewed all cases with LCH between 1968 and 2009 at their center. From the 121 patients, 79 were males and 42 females with a median age of 4.13 years. Three quarters of cases were mono-systemic, and one quarter multi-systemic. The overall survival rate was 93% at 10 years from diagnosis, while the event-free survival was 77%.

The younger age of onset (<2 years) and multi-system involvement were associated with worse prognosis. High risk patients with the involvement of the bone marrow, spleen, liver and lungs had only 50% overall survival in contrast to low risk patients who had 94% overall survival. Fourteen patients developed diabetes insipidus, 7 growth hormone deficiencies, 2 hypothyroidism and 1 neurodegeneration. The overall survival also improved during the later years of the review, reflecting a better therapeutic management (Posini et al., 2012). Cases of spontaneous healing of skin and bone lesions have been reported (Oliveira et al., 2012, Tsai and Tzeng 2012).

The involvement of the central nervous system (CNS) in LCH has been recognized since the early reports of the disease (Schueller 1915, Christian 1920, Hand 1921). CNS changes are typically described either as granulomatous or neurodegenerative lesions. Grois et al. (2005) distinguished three types of the lesions: (a) circumscribed granulomas within the brain's connective tissue space, such as the meninges or choroids plexus (Figure 1. and Figure 2), (b) granulomas within the brain's connective tissue spaces with partial infiltration of surrounding CNS parenchyma, and (c) neurodegenerative lesions.

Granulomatous lesions are composed of CD1a and CD207 (langerin) positive cells admixed with eosinophils, polyclonal CD4+, FoxP3+ T cells, macrophages and osteoclast-like multinucleated giant cells (Satoh et al., 2012). The granulomas may affect various parts of the CNS causing corresponding clinical defects. The pituitary gland is frequently affected associated with diabetes insipidus and growth hormone or other endocrine defects.

Neurodegenerative lesions are less frequent and typically involve the cerebellar white matter, dentate nuclei, brain stem and the basal ganglia. These lesions appear as symmetric hyperintense lesions on T2-weighted magnetic resonance images (MRI), without contrast enhancement on T1-weighted images.

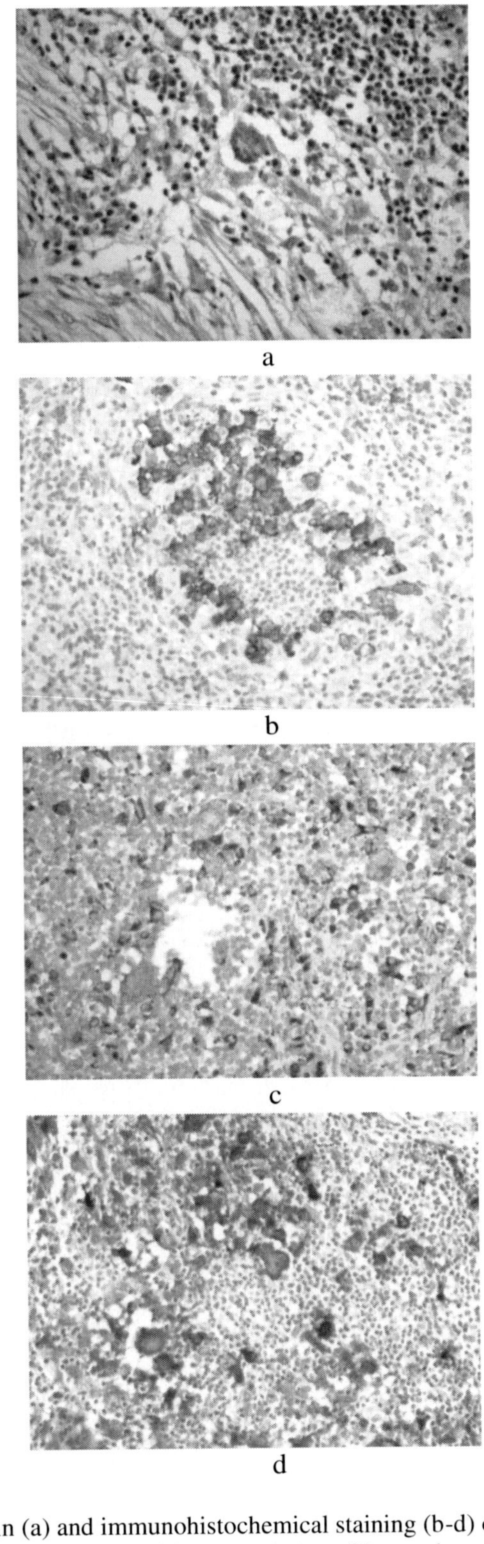

Figure 1. Hematoxylin-eosin (a) and immunohistochemical staining (b-d) of an eosinophil granuloma. Figure 1a shows cellularity of the lesion with accumulation of Langerhans cells (polymorph, foamy histiocytes), multiple eosinophils and a giant cell conglomerate (60x); 1b – CD1a positive cells (20x); 1c – CD68 positive cells (60x); and 1d – S100 positive cells (40x).

Atrophy in the cerebellum and brain stem may also be observed. The pathological correlates of these lesions include demyelination and gliosis in the cerebellar nuclei, brainstem nuclei and cerebellar peduncules, as well as neuronal loss in the Purkinje and granular cell layers in the cerebellum. Occasionally, calcification may also be present in the cerebellar nuclei. CD1a histiocytes are absent while CD8+ cells are conspicuously present, suggesting an inflammatory, possibly paraneoplastic cause of the neurodegenerative process (Ekici et al., 2011, Federico and Di Toro Mammarella 2012). The clinical manifestation depends on the affected CNS regions, and ranges from asymptomatic involvement, through mild tremor and subtle neurological findings, to severe corticospinal, cerebellar, extrapyramidal, brainstem or psychiatric presentations (Federico and Di Toro Mammarella 2012).

The clinical suspicion for diagnosis of histiocytosis is confirmed by immunohistochemistry showing CD1a, S100 and langerin (CD207) positivity of cells in the lesions or by electron microscopy showing the presence of Birbeck granules (Oliveira et al., 2012, Schmitt-Graeff et al., 2012). Figure 1a-d illustrates the typical histological appearance and immunohistochemical characteristics of an eosinophilic granuloma. Routine blood tests are usually non-revealing. Adrenocorticotropic hormone (ACTH), growth hormone (GH), follicle-stimulating hormone (FSH), luteinizing hormone (LH), cortisol, testosterone and thyroid hormone tests may be informative in cases of the pituitary involvement.

The treatment of LCH depends of the spread of pathology and the organ involvement. While isolated cutaneous lesions may spontaneously resolve (Wheller et al., 2013, Yurkovich et al., 2013), most cases require treatment including topical steroids, oral methotrexate or thalidomide. Psoralen and long-wave ultraviolet radiation have also been used with success (Gupta and Bansal 2012). Organ involvement in LCD is usually treated with chemotherapy (methotrexate, etoposide) and irradiation (Lajolo et al., 2012, Kotecha et al., 2013). Long-lasting responses in LCH can be typically achieved by combined and aggressive chemotherapy. Salvage therapy with cytarabine and cladribine also showed promise in the treatment of children with refractory, risk-organ positive LCH, but these agents are associated with significant toxicity. Recent data suggest that in refractory cases clofarabine as a single agent may be an effective alternative treatment with the advantage of minimal toxicity (Abraham et al., 2012). Pituitary involvement requires hormonal replacement, most commonly using desmopressin in diabetes insipidus. Since LCH lesions in the temporal bone often cause conductive or less commonly sensorineural hearing loss, post-labyrinthectomy cochlear implantation may be necessary to restore hearing (Segel and McKinnon, 2013).

Langerhans cells are dendritic cells involved in antigen processing and presentation in epithelial surfaces such as the skin and mucosa, which drive the differentiation or tolerance of antigen specific lymphocytes (Schmitt-Graeff et al., 2012). They have myeloid origin and share common ancestry with monocytes, which is suggested by similar surface antigens in the two lineages during differentiation. As pointed out above, LCH are defined by their CD1a, S100 and CD207 (langerin) positivity. Several lines of observations suggest that LCH may result from a clonal expansion of cells acquiring somatic genomic mutations (Feldman et al., 2004, 2005, 2008, Ratei et al., 2010, Gong et al., 2010). In patients with follicular lymphoma or acute lymphoblastic leukemia / lymphoma of T and B cell lineages, cells with LC surface characteristics have been detected. Identical clonality was supported by the detection of similar T Cell Receptor or Immunoglobulin (Ig)H rearrangements in the leukemia / lymphoma cells and the LC tumor. This observation suggests that a histiocytic / dentritic cell tumor may develop from subclones of lymphoid malignancies (Feldman et al., 2004, 2005, 2008, Ratei et al., 2010, Gong et al., 2010, Schmitt-Graeff et al., 2012). In contrast, LCH followed by Hodgkin's lymphoma was also reported (Park et al., 2012). In addition, association between LCH and acute myeloid leukemia (AML) has been described (Egeler et al., 1994). However, in these cases the development of AML followed the treatment of LCH, suggesting that the AML most likely developed secondary to the LCH treatment (Egeler et al., 1994, Schmitt-Graeff et al., 2012). Further, case reports revealed the co-occurrence of LCH and myeloid sarcoma (MS) characterized by the same chromosomal abnormality (chromosome 8 trisomy), but dichotomous expression of Id2 (a dominant negative helix-loop-helix transcription factor of the ID family) present in the LCs but absent in the MS cells (Pileri et al., 2007, Schmitt-Graeff et al., 2012). This study suggested *in vivo* differentiation of myeloid blast subpopulations into LCH cells with CD1a and langerin expression.

The overall results of investigations as to whether LCH stems from a polyclonal reactivation or from a monoclonal malignant expansion favor today the latter. One of the assays used for the investigation of clonality is the HUMARA assay that defines the random inactivation mosaicism of maternal or paternal X-chromosomes by methylation in a somatic tissue. A highly polymorphic short tandem repeat (CAG) in exon 1 of the human androgen receptor on the X-chromosome has also been tested for evaluating clonality. Using the X-linked polymorphic DNA probes and the HUMARA assay, LCH appeared monoclonal in origin (William et al., 1994, Yu et al., 1994), a finding that does not necessarily signify cancer. Traulsen et al. (2010) discuss three mutations (BCR-ABL, PIG-A and Jak2 genes – characteristics of chronic myeloid leukemia, paroxysmal nocturnal hemoglobulinemia and myeloproliferative disease, respectively) to demonstrate that the population frequencies of these disorders fit in the hierarchical model of hematopoiesis, and the fate of a mutant clone depends on the target cell and the fitness advantage of the mutation conferred on the cell. The authors propose that mutations in a hematopoietic stem cell will lead to long-lasting hematological disease or malignancy, while mutations affecting non-stem cells cause less severe somatic perturbations.

In the context of acquired molecular abnormalities, it is important noting that mutations observed in cancer may also be present in LCH, without signs of malignancy. B-RAF protein kinase somatic mutations (V600E) were reported in 57% of LCH granuloma cells (Badalian-Very et al., 2010). This finding was confirmed and expanded by Satoh et al. (2012), showing not only the presence of the ^{V600E}B-RAF mutation, but also the presence of two additional B-RAF mutations in the granuloma of 11 of their 16 patients, who harbored no such mutations in their blood. The RAS-RAF-MAPK signaling pathway represents a key communication line involved in cell-cycle, proliferation, differentiation, survival and apoptosis, by mediating extracellular signals to intracellular responder elements bound to membranes and localized to the cytoplasm or the nucleus (Satoh et al., 2012).

Expression of the ^{V600E}B-RAF in mice showed that this mutation can induce tumor development (Pritchard et al., 2007), while it has also been detected in a number of benign and malignant human tumors including melanoma, nevi, papillary thyroid carcinoma, colorectal cancer, hairy cell leukemia and non-small cell lung cancer (Pollock et al., 2003, Dankort et al., 2009). It appears that the occurrence of ^{V600E}B-RAF may be a step towards tumor development, but the presence of this mutation alone does not necessarily signify malignant transformation (Satoh et al., 2012).

Accumulation of additional, so called "driver" mutations (affecting key regulators of cell cycle, proliferation, DNA repair, apoptosis, etc…) likely define the overall cell behavior and a malignant phenotype. This is in line with the above discussed concept proposed by Traulsen et al. (2010) and with the notion that LCH does not qualify for cancer as its proliferation rate is low, the lesions may regress or respond well to treatment (Satoh et al., 2012).

Nevertheless, the identification of the outlined molecular pathways and mutations, places LCH in the proximity of hematological malignancies, and call for a close hematological monitoring of patients who present with LCH. These molecular findings also represent an important step forward to better understand the disease pathogenesis and have lead to the identification of vemurafenib, a B-RAF inhibitor, as a potential new treatment modality in LCH. Vemurafenib, approved for the treatment of ^{V600E}B-RAF positive melanoma, also appeared effective in the treatment of severe and refractory LCH (Haroche et al., 2013). Multi-dimensional (genomic, transcriptomic, proteomic, epigenomic) and longitudinal analyses of the LCH lesions may help to gain further insights into the generation of this serious, but by definition non-malignant condition (Landi et al., 2013).

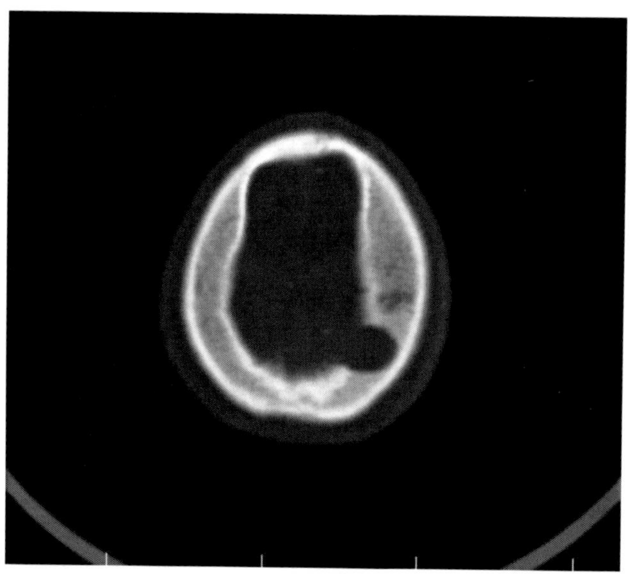

Figure 2. Imaging of an eosinophil granuloma. The axial non-enhanced computer tomography scan of the skull with an osteolytic lesion at the calvarium shows destruction in the inner tablet of the skull expanding into the diploic space. Histology work up (shown in Figure 1) verified the lesion as an eosinophil granuloma.

2. Erdheim-Chester Disease (ECD)

ECD was described as a disorder with lipoid granulomatosis by William Chester (1930), Jakob Erdheim´s pupil. In 1972, Jaffe reported a similar case and coined the term of Erdheim-Chester disease (Jaffe, 1972). Since then until July 2011, 445 cases had been reported, reflecting the rarity of the disease (Haroche et al., 2012). The number of cases, however, started to somewhat increase in recent years, due to more sensitive imaging techniques, better immune-molecular definition of the cellular pathology and a wider recognition of the entity.

Haroche et al. (2012) reviewed characteristics of their 75 patients, and reported 73% male and 27% female involvement. As opposed to LHC that is typically a pediatric disorder, ECD primarily (although not exclusively) affects adults with a mean age of onset at 55+/-14 years (range 16-80 years).

ECD is a non-LC histiocytosis, a systemic disease that may also affect multiple organs including the long bones, skin, kidneys, retroperitoneum, lungs, the wall of the heart and the pericardium, extra-axial and intra-axial parts of the CNS, the pituitary and the retro-orbital regions (Haroche et al., 2012). The prognosis of ECD depends on the extent of pathology and the involvement of internal organs and the CNS. The clinical pictures range from asymptomatic, through subtle symptomatic to severe life-threatening presentations.

The extent of the disease may be assessed by multi-modal imaging techniques including technetium-99 (^{99}Tc) bone scintigraphy, 18F-fluoro-desoxy-glucose – positron emission tomography (PET) scan, computer tomography (CT), organ-specific or whole body (WB)-MRI (Arnaud et al., 2012).

Almost all ECD patients have skeletal involvement that usually presents with mild bone pain in half of the patients, and predominantly in the lower extremities. Radiographs show bilateral and symmetric cortical osteosclerosis in the diaphyseal and metaphyseal regions (Figure 3), while tracer uptake in ^{99}Tc-bone scintigraphy can be seen in the long bones in almost all cases (Haroche et al., 2012).

In contrast to LCH, the axial skeleton and flat bones are rarely involved in ECD (Wilejto 2012). The vertebral and mandibular bones are usually (though not always) spared. The involvements of the orbital and retro-orbital region may cause painless exophthalmos (Wilejto 2012) and optic nerve impairment.

Cutaneous lesions were seen in 28% of the 53 patients by Haroches et al. (2012), and included xanthelasmas preferentially in the eyelids or in the periorbital spaces, papulonodular lesions and genital (vulva and clitoris) infiltrations.

Among cardiovascular lesions, the most frequent involvement is the circumferential periaortic sheathing of the abdominal and thoracic aorta (coated aorta), which can also extend to the main aortic branches (Figure 4). While this sheathing may remain asymptomatic, the involvement of renal arteries is associated with hypertension manageable by stenting (Haroche et al., 2012, Alexiev and Staats, 2013). The infiltration around the coronary arteries may lead to myocardial infarction. Another life threatening cardiac complication is the cardiac tamponade caused by pericardial infiltration which was detected in 42% of the reviewed 53 patients by Haroche et al. (2012). Myocardial, endocardial and valvular involvements less frequently occur. The histiocytic infiltration may extend to any of the visceral organs, but only rarely noted in the gastro-intestinal system (Pan et al., 2011).

Pseudo "retroperitoneal fibrosis" was reported in 30% of patients with ECD (Haroche et al., 2012), often complicated with ureteral stenosis and hydronephrosis, which are also manageable by stenting. However, the pelvic ureters and the vena cava are typically spared in ECD, as opposed to that seen in idiopathic retroperitoneal fibrosis. The authors also reported a "hairy kidney" appearance on abdominal CT in about 50% of their 53 cases (Haroche et al., 2012) (Figure 4).

Pulmonary involvement is common in ECD, but appears to influence the prognosis to a lesser degree than the involvement of the cardiovascular system. High resolution chest CT revealed parenchymal involvement in 53% and pleural involvement in 41% in 34 patients with ECD (Brun et al., 2010, Haroche et al., 2012).

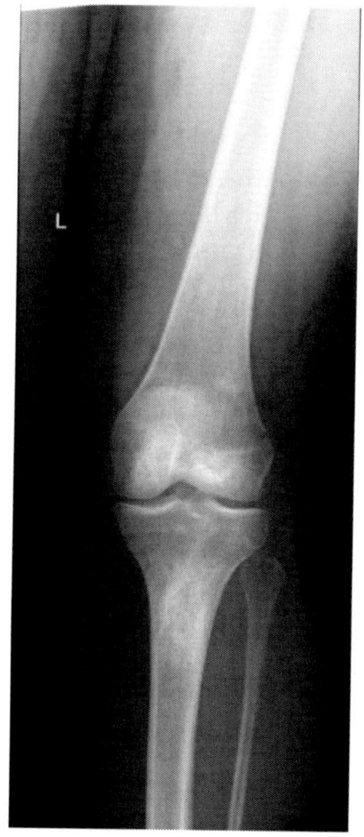

Figure 3. Conventional radiograph of the left knee of a patient with ECD. The radiograph shows bone involvement, where there is inhomogeneous osteosclerosis in the proximal metaphysis of the tibia, which turned out to be bilateral.

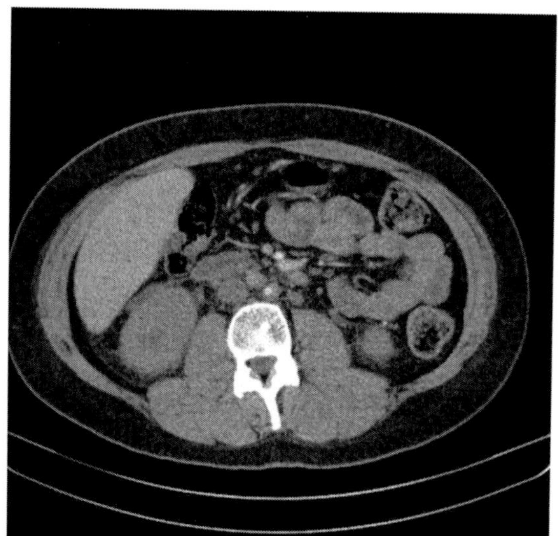

Figure 4. Abdominal computer tomography scan of a patient with ECD. The axial computer tomography scan acquired in arterial phase after intravenous iodine contrast medium administration shows severe reduction of the aortic lumen ("coated aorta") and perirenal infiltration ("hairy kidney appearance") in a patient with ECD.

In addition to pericardial and pleural effusion, perirenal soft-tissue abnormalities (hairy kidney) and osteosclerotic lesions of the tibia, and massive ascites were also reported in an elderly patient with ECD (Ota et al., 2013).

The involvement of the CNS is a major negative prognostic factor and independent predictor of death in ECD (Arnaud et al., 2011, Haroche et al., 2012, Cavalli et al., 2013). CNS involvement occurs in about 15-25% of cases (Lachenal et al., 2006). Most frequently, signs of corticospinal and cerebellar involvements are seen, but diabetes insipidus and/or anterior pituitary hormone deficiency, sensory abnormalities, cranial nerve lesions, headaches, seizures, cognitive deterioration, exophthalmos, and psychiatric presentations also occur (Figure 5).

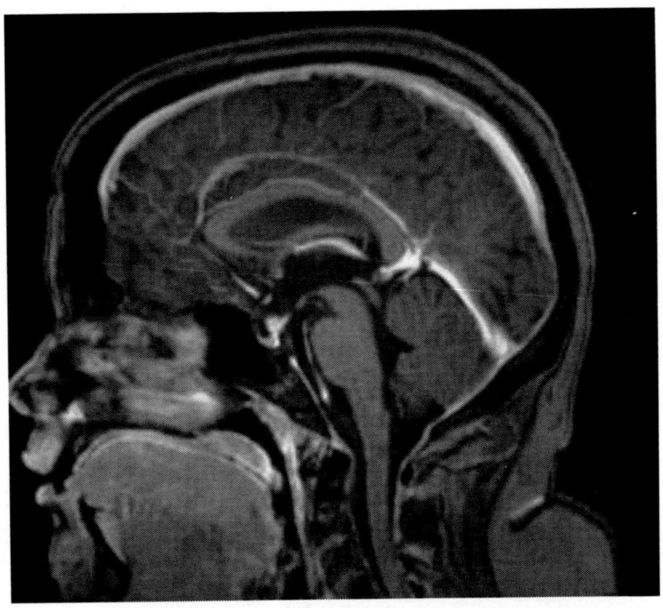

Figure 5. 3T T1-weighted, contrast-enhanced brain MRI of a patient with ECD. The image shows the widening of the hypophyseal infundibulum. The patient suffered from diabetes insipidus.

The pathology may involve the brain parenchyma, meninges, retro-orbital and pituitary regions (Haroche et al., 2012, Sharma et al., 2013). On imaging, parenchymal brain lesions may mimic multiple sclerosis. In addition, intra-cranial extra-axial lesions with stellate appearance, ependymal enhancement along the lateral ventricle and deep linear extension to the lentiform nucleus, irregular enhancement in the pons and diffuse involvement of the vertebral columns were reported using CT, MRI and PET/CT (Sedrak et al., 2011).

The ultimate histological confirmation of the clinical diagnosis of ECD depends on the result of immunohistochemistry demonstrating CD68+ and CD1a- foamy histiocytes in polymorphic granulomatous and fibrotic or xanthogranulomatous lesions (as opposed to CD1a+ cells in lesions of LCH) (Figure 6a-d). The S100 staining is variable. ECD is associated with systemic immune activation and altered cytokine / chemokine production (interleukin [IL]-1, interferon [IFN]-α, IL-6, IL-12, monocyte chemotactic protein [MCP]-1) (Haroche et al., 2012). Elevated level of IL-6 likely plays a role in aberrant bone turnover, and causes osteosclerosis (Wilejto et al. 2012).

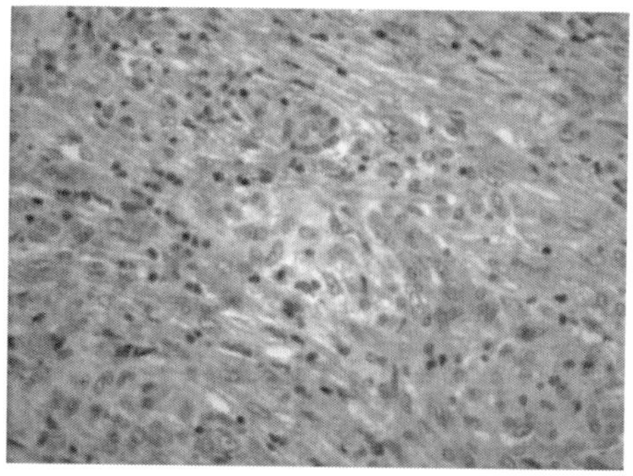

a

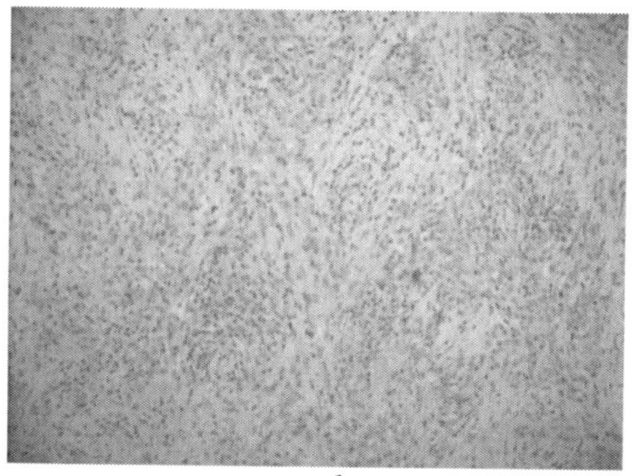

b

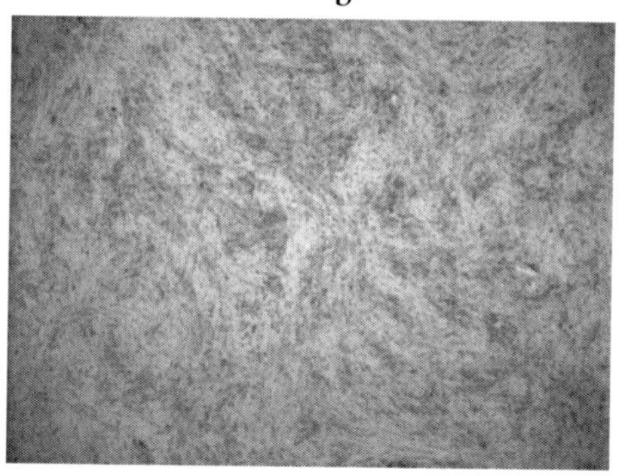

c

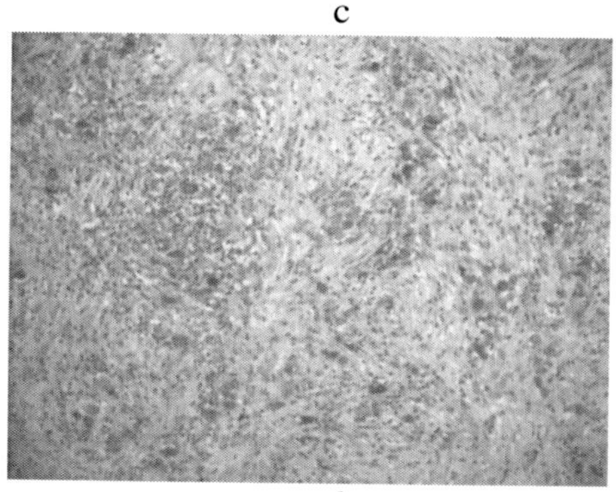

d

Figure 6. Hematoxylin-eosin (a) and immunohistochemical (b-d) staining of a lesion from a patient with ECD. Figure 6a shows polymorph, foamy macrophages (histiocytes) and a cellular conglomerate forming a giant cell in a fibrotic lesion (60x); 6b – CD1a negative cells (20x); 3c – CD68 positive cells (20x); and 6d – S100 positive cells (40x).

Several treatment modalities have been used for ECD, which include steroids, cladribine, IFN-α, recombinant IL-1 receptor antagonists, thyrosine kinase inhibitors, and autologous hemopoietic cell transplantation (Arnaud et al., 2011). While the use of these modalities is not supported by the results of double-blind, randomized and placebo-controlled trials, a recent multi-center, prospective and observational study revealed positive findings in patients with extra-skeletal manifestations of ECD and IFN-α treatment (Arnaud et al., 2011). Survival analyses were performed in 53 biopsy-proven patients with ECD followed between November 1981 and November 2010.

During this period, 46 patients (87%) received IFN-α and/or pegylated IFN-α. Multivariate survival analysis using Cox proportional hazard model showed that the involvement of CNS was an independent predictor of death (hazard ratio = 2.51; 95% confidence interval, 1.28-5.52; p= 0.006), while IFN-α treatment was an independent predictor of survival (hazard ratio = 0.32; 95% confidence interval, 0.14-0.70; p= 0.006). This study strongly supports the benefit of IFN-α treatment in ECD (Haroche et al., 2004, Arnaud et al., 2011). Subsequently, the use of IFN-α in ECD received further support (Hervier et al., 2012). In this study, 24 patients with CNS or cardiac involvement or exophthalmos and failure to standard (9 mIU/week) IFN-α treatment received high dose IFN-α =/> 18 mIU/week or pegylated IFN-α =/> 180 ug/week, with a median follow up of 19 months using clinical and imaging evaluation for outcome. High dose IFN-α treatment resulted in improvement in 16 (67%), and stabilization in 5 (21%) of the patients.

Among patients with CNS involvement, improvement was noted in 7/11 (64%) and among those with cardiac involvement the improvement rate was 11/14 (79%). Six patients (25%) worsened. High dose IFN-α was well tolerated, and despite some side effects (asthenia, pruritus, myalgia, thrombocytopenia, depression), the drop-out rate was low. This study further underscored the importance of IFN-α, particularly high-dose IFN-α, in the management of ECD. Generally, pegylated IFN-α and / or IFN-α is considered as first line treatment for ECD today, and recommended in high doses (180 ug/week or 18-27 mIU/week, respectively, divided into three administrations per week). This treatment is given in long duration, particularly for patients with cardiovascular and CNS involvement. The mechanisms through which this pleiotropic cytokine may exert its beneficial effects include an impact on the differentiation of dendritic cells, enhancement of the activity of the natural killer cells targeting histiocytes, and a direct anti-proliferative effect (Haroche et al., 2012).

The benefit of IFN-α in ECD is also supported by the comparison of data from two consecutive survival analyses. In the first study, 35 of 58 patients (60%) died with a mean survival time of 19.2 months after the diagnosis (Haroche et al., 2004). This study preceded the use of IFN-α in ECD. In the second study, a significant decrease in mortality (15%) was found after treatment with IFN-α (Arnaud et al., 2011). The 5-year survival rate was 68% in this report.

The underlying cellular and molecular abnormality of ECD is less clear than that of LCH. Occasionally, the two rare conditions can be observed simultaneously and even in the same tissue distribution (Pineles et al. 2011, Yin et al., 2013). This intra-individual clustering of LCH and ECD may be explained by a common progenitor (CD34) of the CD1a+, CD207+, CD68+ and the CD1a-, CD68+ lineages (Pineles et al., 2011). The existence of a common progenitor is further supported by successful therapeutic intervention in LCH and ECD using imatinib mesylate (Gleevec® or Glivec®, Novartis Inc.) that can act on CD34+ peripheral blood progenitor cells, inhibit their differentiation to dendritic cells, and thereby inhibit the activation of lymphocytes (Janku et al., 2010).

Both clinical and imaging evaluations showed marked improvement on this regimen in two patients with LCH and one patient with ECD. Imatinib is a competitive inhibitor of protein kinases associated with the ABL, ARG, KIT, PDGFRA and PDGFRB signaling molecules. Imatinib is approved by the US Food and Drug Administration (FDA) for the treatment of several hematological malignancies and solid tumors with function-gaining rearrangements that affect some of the listed protein kinases. The beneficial effect of imatinib may be explained by its inhibition of PDGFRB that is often expressed in both LCH and ECD, although mutations causing constitutive PDGFRB expression have not been identified in either one of the two conditions (Janku et al., 2012).

In addition, Haroche et al. (2013) reported three patients with systemic and refractory ECD carrying the ^{V600E}B-RAF mutation. All patients responded dramatically to the B-RAF inhibitor, vemurafenib, and the responses were sustained for several months (Haroche et al., 2013). As 54% of patients with ECD carry the ^{V600E}B-RAF mutation, vemurafenib or related inhibitors of the RAF-RAS-MAPK signaling pathway may represent an effective treatment of selected patients with ECD (Haroche et al., 2013).

The question of monoclonal expansion as opposed to polyclonal reactivation arose in ECD similar to that in LCH. The results of investigations, however, remain less conclusive in ECD when testing with the HUMARA assay that demonstrated both polyclonal and monoclonal patterns in ECD lesions in various studies (Al-Quran et al., 2002, Chetritt et al., 1999, Gong et al., 2009). Monoclonal expansion of CD68+ and CD1a- / S100- cells in a tibial tumor, however, also have been demonstrated with a balanced chromosomal translocation t(12;15;20)(q11;q24;p13.3) (Vencio et al., 2007). These mixed findings may reflect technical difficulties (e.g., the separation of non-LC histiocytes from the "diluting" organ specific or inflammatory cells) or a biological heterogeneity of the disease, and highlight the need to comprehensively reinvestigate the lesions by using newer methods of molecular genetics.

3. Rosai-Dorfman Disease

Rosai-Dorfman disease (RDD) is a sinus histiocytosis with lymphadenopathy. RDD was first described in 1969 by Juan Rosai and Ronald Dorfman in a young black male (Rosai et al. 1969). Histiocytes in this condition bear similar characteristics to histiocytes seen in ECD, but emperipolesis (phagocytosis) of lymphocytes by these cells have been described (Al-Quran et al., 2002). These histiocytes are immunhistochemically positive for S100 and CD68, and negative for CD1a. RDD affects children and young adults with a mean age of 20.6 years and with male predominance (Mahzoni et al. 2012).

The presentation typically includes bilateral, painless, and massive cervical lymphadenopathy. Extranodal involvement is documented in 43% of the patients, occasionally accompanied with lymphadenopathy early or later in the disease. The most common extranodal involvements include the skin, nasal cavity, paranasal sinuses, eyelids, orbits, bones, salivary glands and the CNS. The CNS is affected in less than 5% of RDD cases.

In 70% of CNS-RDD, the presentation is limited to the brain (75%) or to the spinal cord (25%) and is not associated with lymphadenopathy (Roy et al., 2012). Over 90% of CNS RDD, the leptomeninges are only involved (Mahzoni et al. 2012). Intracranial RDD often mimics meningioma in radiographic appearances and it may still be challenging to differentiate between these two diseases. It is worth noting, however, that calcification has not been reported in RDD. The diagnosis of RDD primarily relies on histological and immunohistochemical findings (Tomio et al. 2012). Its molecular etiology remains unclear, but infectious origin and abnormal Fas / Fas ligand signaling have been implicated (Mahzoni et al., 2012).

Overall, RDD has a good prognosis, although it may also have severe presentations. Spontaneous remission was reported in 20% of patients, and about 50% of patients did not need any treatments. Common treatment modalities include surgery, steroids, chemotherapeutic agents and radiation. Surgical resection and radiotherapy seem to be the most effective treatments in life-threatening disease with rapid progression in the lymph node (Noguchi et al. 2012, Setareh et al., 2013).

Conclusion

Histiocytosis remains a rare and partially understood entity with a great proportion of cases having neurological involvement. The *in vivo* diagnostic identification has significantly increased during the last few years due to improved imaging and histological work up. As the underlying molecular pathogeneses of both CD1a+ and CD1a- histiocyte lineages are better understood, and the availability of both pleiotropic and single-molecule targeting therapeutic modalities is increasing, the prognosis of LCH, ECD and RDD is steadily improving. Further explorations of the acquired somatic abnormalities in histiocytic lineages will enable us to better understand disease pathogenesis and get closer to the cure of this clinically highly variable entity.

References

Abraham A, Alsultan A, Jeng M, Rodriguez-Galindo C, Campbell PK. Clofarabine salvage therapy for refractory high-risk langerhans cell histiocytosis. *Pediatr. Blood Cancer.* 2012 Dec 19. doi: 10.1002/pbc.24436. [Epub ahead of print].

Alexiev BA, Staats PN. Erdheim-Chester Disease With Prominent Pericardial Effusion: Cytologic Findings and Review of the Literature. *Diagn. Cytopathol.* 2013 Feb 28. doi: 10.1002/dc.22957. [Epub ahead of print]

Al-Quran S, Reith J, Bradley J, Rimsza L.Erdheim.Chester Disease: Case report, PCR-based analysis of clonality, and review of literature. *Mol. Pathol.* 2002;15(6)666-672.

Arico M, Girschikofsky M, Genereau T et al.: Langerhans cell histiocytosis in adults. *Eur. J. Cancer* 2003; 39:2341-2348.

Arnaud L, Bach G, Zeitoun D, Drier A, Cluzel P, Grenier PA, Amoura Z, Haroche J. Whole-body MRI in Erdheim-Chester disease. *Rheumatology* (Oxford). 2012 May;51(5):948-50. Epub 2012 Feb 29.

Arnaud L, Hervier B, Néel A, Hamidou MA, Kahn JE, Wechsler B, Pérez-Pastor G, Blomberg B, Fuzibet JG, Dubourguet F, Marinho A, Magnette C, Noel V, Pavic M, Casper J, Beucher AB, Costedoat-Chalumeau N, Aaron L, Salvatierra J, Graux C, Cacoub P, Delcey V, Dechant C, Bindi P, Herbaut C, Graziani G, Amoura Z, Haroche J. CNS involvement and treatment with interferon-α are independent prognostic factors in Erdheim-Chester disease: a multicenter survival analysis of 53 patients. *Blood.* 2011 Mar 10;117(10):2778-82. Epub 2011 Jan 14.

Badalian-Very G, Vergilio JA, Degar BA, MacConaill LE, Brandner B, Calicchio ML, Kuo FC, Ligon AH, Stevenson KE, Kehoe SM, Garraway LA, Hahn WC, Meyerson M, Fleming MD, Rollins BJ. Recurrent BRAF mutations in Langerhans cell histiocytosis. *Blood.* 2010 Sep 16;116(11):1919-23. Epub 2010 Jun 2.

Badalian-Very G, Vergilio JA, Degar BA, Rodriguez-Galindo C, Rollins BJ. Recent advances in the understanding of Langerhans cell histiocytosis. *Br. J. Haematol.* 2012 Jan;156(2):163-72. doi: 10.1111/j.1365-2141.2011.08915.x. Epub 2011 Oct 24.

Brun AL, Touitou-Gottenberg D, Haroche J, Toledano D, Cluzel P, Beigelman-Aubry C, Piette JC, Amoura Z, Grenier PA. Erdheim-Chester disease: CT findings of thoracic involvement. *Eur. Radiol.* 2010 Nov;20(11):2579-87. Epub 2010 Jun 20.

Cavalli G, Guglielmi B, Berti A, Campochiaro C, Sabbadini MG, Dagna L. The multifaceted clinical presentations and manifestations of Erdheim-Chester disease: comprehensive review of the literature and of 10 new cases. *Ann. Rheum. Dis.* 2013 Feb 8. [Epub ahead of print]

Chester W. Uber lipidgranulomatose. *Virchows Arch. A Pathol. Anat. Histol.* 1930;279:561-602.

Chetrott J, Paradis V, Dargere D, Adle-Biasette H, Maurage CA, Mussini JM, et al. Chester-Erdheim disease: a neoplastic disorder. *Hum. Pathol.* 1999;30:1093-6.

Dankort D, Curley DP, Cartlidge RA, Nelson B, Karnezis AN, Damsky WE Jr, You MJ, DePinho RA, McMahon M, Bosenberg M. Braf(V600E) cooperates with Pten loss to induce metastatic melanoma. *Nat. Genet.* 2009 May;41(5):544-52. Epub 2009 Mar 12.

Egeler RM, Neglia JP, Aricò M, Favara BE, Heitger A, Nesbit ME. Acute leukemia in association with Langerhans cell histiocytosis. *Med. Pediatr. Oncol.* 1994;23(2):81-5.

Ekici B, Gümüş S, Ozmen M, Devecioğlu O. Histiocytosis-related cerebellar leukoencephalopathy. *J. Pediatr Neurosci.* 2011 Jul;6(2):162-3.

Federico A and Di Toro Mammarella L. Progressive neurodegenerative syndrome associated with Langerhans cell histiocytosis: a rare condition that we have to consider in patients with sporadic spastic ataxia and diabetes insipidus. *Neur. Sci.* 2012;33:489-490.

Feldman AL, Minniti C, Santi M, Downing JR, Raffeld M, Jaffe ES. Histiocytic sarcoma after acute lymphoblastic leukaemia: a common clonal origin. *Lancet Oncol.* 2004 Apr;5(4):248-50.

Feldman AL, Berthold F, Arceci RJ, Abramowsky C, Shehata BM, Mann KP, Lauer SJ, Pritchard J, Raffeld M, Jaffe ES. Clonal relationship between precursor T-lymphoblastic leukaemia/lymphoma and Langerhans-cell histiocytosis. *Lancet Oncol.* 2005 Jun;6(6):435-7.

Feldman AL, Arber DA, Pittaluga S, Martinez A, Burke JS, Raffeld M, Camos M, Warnke R, Jaffe ES. Clonally related follicular lymphomas and histiocytic/dendritic cell sarcomas: evidence for transdifferentiation of the follicular lymphoma clone. *Blood.* 2008 Jun 15;111(12):5433-9.

Gong L, He XL, Li YH, Ren KX, Zhang L, Liu XY, Han XJ, Yao L, Zhu SJ, Lan M, Zhang W. Clonal status and clinicopathological feature of Erdheim-Chester disease. *Pathol. Res. Pract.* 2009;205(9):601-7. Epub 2009 Apr 1.

Gong L, Zhang WD, Li YH, Liu XY, Yao L, Han XJ, Zhu SJ, Lan M, Zhang W. Clonal status and clinicopathological features of Langerhans cell histiocytosis. *J. Int. Med. Res.* 2010 May-Jun;38(3):1099-105.

Gupta V and Bansal M. Cutaneous Langerhans Cell Histiocytosis. *Indian Pediatrics* 2012;49:79.

Grois N, Prayer D, Prosch H, Lassmann H and the CNS LCH Co-operative Gloup. Neuropathology of CNS disease in Langerhans cell histiocytosis. *Brain*, 2005, 128:829-838.

Haroche J, Arnaud L, Amoura Z. Erdheim-Chester disease. *Curr. Opin. Rheumatol.* 2012 Jan;24(1):53-9. Review.

Haroche J, Cohen-Aubart F, Emile JF, Arnaud L, Maksud P, Charlotte F, Cluzel P, Drier A, Hervier B, Benameur N, Besnard S, Donadieu J, Amoura Z. Dramatic efficacy of vemurafenib in both multisystemic and refractory Erdheim-Chester disease and Langerhans cell histiocytosis harboring the BRAF V600E mutation. *Blood.* 2013 Feb 28;121(9):1495-500.

Hervier B, Arnaud L, Charlotte F, Wechsler B, Piette JC, Amoura Z, Haroche J. Treatment of Erdheim-Chester Disease with Long-Term High-Dose Interferon-α. *Semin Arthritis Rheum.* 2012 Jun;41(6):907-13. Epub 2012 Jan 31.

Jaffe HL. Gaucher´s disease and certain other inborn metabolic disorders: lipid (cholesterol) granulomatosis. In: Jaffe HL, ed. *Metabolic and inflammatory disease of the bone and joints.* Philadelphia, PA: Lea & Febiger; 1972. p. 535-41.

Janku F, Amin HM, Yang D, Garrido-Laguna I, Trent JC, Kurzrock R. Response of histiocytoses to imatinib mesylate: fire to ashes. *J. Clin. Oncol.* 2010 Nov 1;28(31):e633-6. Epub 2010 Aug 23.

Kotecha R, Venkatramani R, Jubran RF, Arkader A, Olch AJ, Wong K. Clinical Outcomes of Radiation Therapy in the Management of Langerhans Cell Histiocytosis. *Am. J. Clin. Oncol.* 2013 Mar 4. [Epub ahead of print]

Lachenal F, Cotton F, Desmurs-Clavel H, Haroche J, Taillia H, Magy N, Hamidou M, Salvatierra J, Piette JC, Vital-Durand D, Rousset H. Neurological manifestations and neuroradiological presentation of Erdheim-Chester disease: report of 6 cases and systematic review of the literature. *J. Neurol.* 2006 Oct;253(10):1267-77. Epub 2006 Oct 24. Review.

Lajolo C, Campisi G, Deli G, Littarru C, Guiglia R, Giuliani M. Langerhans's cell histiocytosis in old subjects: two rare case reports and review of the literature. *Gerodontology.* 2012 Jun;29(2):e1207-14.

Landi C, Bargagli E, Bianchi L, Gagliardi A, Carleo A, Bennet D, Perari MG, Armini A, Prasse A, Rottoli P, Bini L. Towards a functional proteomics approach to the comprehension of idiopathic pulmonary fibrosis, sarcoidosis, systemic sclerosis and pulmonary Langerhans cell histiocytosis. *J. Proteomics.* 2013 Mar 23. doi:pii: S1874-3919(13)00145-0. 10.1016/j.jprot.2013.03.006 [Epub ahead of print].

Lichtenstein L. Histiocytosis X; integration of eosinophilic granuloma of bone, Letterer-Siwe disease, and Schüller-Christian disease as related manifestations of a single nosologic entity. *AMA Arch. Pathol.* 1953 Jul;56(1):84-102.

Mahzoni P, Zavareh MH, Bagheri M, Hani N, Moqtader B. Intracranial ROSAI-DORFMAN Disease. *J. Res. Med. Sci.* 2012 Mar;17(3):304-7.

Noguchi S, Yatera K, Shimajiri S, Inoue N, Nagata S, Nishida C, Kawanami T, Ishimoto H, Sasaguri Y, Mukae H. Intrathoracic Rosai-Dorfman disease with spontaneous remission: a clinical report and a review of the literature. *Tohoku J. Exp. Med.* 2012;227(3):231-325.

Oliveira A, Pinto de Almeida T, Lobo I, Machado S, Selores M. Langerhans cell histiocytosis: two clinical presentations in the same patient. *Dermatol. Online J.* 2012 Jan 15;18(1):8.

Ota M, Sakamoto M, Sato K, Yoshida Y, Funakubo Asanuma Y, Akiyama Y, Yamakawa M, Mimura T. Immunopathological analysis of Erdheim-Chester disease with massive ascites. *Intern Med.* 2012;51(19):2825-30. Epub 2012 Oct 1.

Pan A, Doyle T, Schlup M, Lubcke R, Schultz M. Unusual manifestation of Erdheim-Chester disease. *BMC Gastroenterol.* 2011 Jun 22;11:77.

Park IS, Park IK, Kim EK, Kim S, Jeon SR, Huh JR, Suh CW. Langerhans cell histiocytosis followed by Hodgkin's lymphoma. *Korean J. Intern Med.* 2012 Dec;27(4):459-62.

Pileri SA, Ascani S, Cox MC, Campidelli C, Bacci F, Piccioli M, Piccaluga PP, Agostinelli C, Asioli S, Novero D, Bisceglia M, Ponzoni M, Gentile A, Rinaldi P, Franco V, Vincelli D, Pileri A Jr, Gasbarra R, Falini B, Zinzani PL, Baccarani M. Myeloid sarcoma: clinico-pathologic, phenotypic and cytogenetic analysis of 92 adult patients. *Leukemia.* 2007 Feb;21(2):340-50.

Pineles SL, Liu GT, Acebes X, Arruga J, Nasta S, Glaser R, Pramick M, Fogt F, Roux PL, Gausas RE. Presence of Erdheim-Chester disease and Langerhans cell histiocytosis in the same patient: a report of 2 cases. *J. Neuroophthalmol.* 2011 Sep;31(3):217-23.

Pollock PM, Harper UL, Hansen KS, Yudt LM, Stark M, Robbins CM, Moses TY, Hostetter G, Wagner U, Kakareka J, Salem G, Pohida T, Heenan P, Duray P, Kallioniemi O, Hayward NK, Trent JM, Meltzer PS. High frequency of BRAF mutations in nevi. *Nat. Genet.* 2003 Jan;33(1):19-20. Epub 2002 Nov 25.

Postini AM, Del Frever AB, Pagano M, Rivetti E, Berger M, Asaftei SD, Barat V. Andreacchio A, Fagioli F. Langerhans cell histiocytosis: 40 years´experience. *J. Pediatr Hematol. Oncol.* 2012 May 22. Epub ahead of print.

Pritchard C, Carragher L, Aldridge V, Giblett S, Jin H, Foster C, Andreadi C, Kamata T. Mouse models for BRAF-induced cancers. *Biochem. Soc. Trans.* 2007 Nov;35(Pt 5):1329-33.

Ratei R, Hummel M, Anagnostopoulos I, Jähne D, Arnold R, Dörken B, Mathas S, Benter T, Dudeck O, Ludwig WD, Stein H. Common clonal origin of an acute B-lymphoblastic leukemia and a Langerhans' cell sarcoma: evidence for hematopoietic plasticity. *Haematologica.* 2010 Sep;95(9):1461-6.

Rosai J, Dorfman R.F. Sinus histiocytosis with massive lymphadenopathy. A newly recognized benign clinicopathological entity. *Arch. Pathol.* 1969:87:63-70.

Roy C, Saha A, Roy S, Ghosh A. Extranodal Rosai-Dorfman Disease presenting as spinal extradural lesion: a case report with a review of the literature. *J. Cancer Res. Ther.* 2012 Oct-Dec;8(4):647-9. doi: 10.4103/0973-1482.106588.

Satoh T, Smith A, Sarde A, Lu HC, Mian S, Trouillet C, Mufti G, Emile JF, Fraternali F, Donadieu J, Geissmann F. B-RAF mutant alleles associated with Langerhans cell histiocytosis, a granulomatous pediatric disease. *PLoS One.* 2012;7(4):e33891. Epub 2012 Apr 10.

Sharma M, Vettiyil B, Bartlett E, Yu E. Suprasellar non-Langerhans cell histiocytosis (Erdheim-Chester disease)-a case report. *Clin. Imaging*. 2013 Mar;37(2):354-7. doi: 10.1016/j.clinimag.2012.06.006. Epub 2012 Jul 15.

Schmitt-Graeff AH, Duerkop H, Vollmer-Kary B, Haxelmans S, Nitschke R, Fisch P, Germing U, Stein H. Clonal relationship between langerhans cell histiocytosis and myeloid sarcoma. *Leukemia*. 2012 Feb 3. doi: 10.1038/leu.2012.27 [Epub ahead of print].

Sedrak P, Ketonen L, Hou P, Guha-Thakurta N, Williams MD, Kurzrock R, Debnam JM. Erdheim-Chester disease of the central nervous system: new manifestations of a rare disease. *AJNR Am. J. Neuroradiol*. 2011 Dec;32(11):2126-31. Epub 2011 Sep 29.

Segel JM, McKinnon BJ. Bilateral cochlear implantation in bilateral Langerhans cell histiocytosis. *Cochlear Implants Int*. 2013 Feb 19 [Epub ahead of print].

Setareh M, Zahra M, Vahid M, Farah S. Generalized lymphadenopathy in infancy; a case report. *Iran J. Pediatr*. 2013 Feb;23(1):105-8.

Stålemark H, Laurencikas E, Karis J, Gavhed D, Fadeel B, Henter JI. Incidence of Langerhans cell histiocytosis in children: a population-based study. *Pediatr Blood* Cancer. 2008 Jul;51(1):76-81.

Tomio R, Katayama M, Takenaka N, Imanishi T. Complications of surgical treatment of Rosai-Dorfman disease: A case report and review. *Surg. Neurol. Int*. 2012;3:1

Traulsen A, Pacheco JM, Luzzatto L, Dingli D. *Somatic mutations and the hierarchy of hematopoiesis. Bioessays*. 2010 Nov;32(11):1003-8. doi: 10.1002/bies.201000025. Epub 2010 Aug 27.

Tsai PY and Tzeng WS. Vertebra Plana with Spontaneous Healing. *New Eng. J. Med.* 2012;366e30.

Vencio EF, Jenkins RB, Schiller JL, Huynh TV, Wenger DD, Inwards CY, Oliveira AM. Clonal cytogenetic abnormalities in Erdheim-Chester disease. *Am. J. Surg. Pathol.* 2007 Feb;31(2):319-21.

Wheller L, Carman N, Butler G. Unilesional self-limited Langerhans cell histiocytosis: a case report and review of the literature. *J. Cutan Pathol.* 2013 Feb 26. doi: 10.1111/cup.12121 Epub ahead of print

Wilejto M, Abla O. Langerhans cell histiocytosis and Erdheim-Chester disease. *Curr. Opin. Rheumatol*. 2012:24:90-96

Writing Group of the Histiocyte Society. Histiocytosis syndromes in children. *Lancet* 1987:24;1(8526):208-9.

Yin J, Zhang F, Zhang H, Shen L, Li Q, Hu S, Tian Q, Bao Y, Jia W. Hand-Schüller-Christian disease and Erdheim-Chester disease: coexistence and discrepancy. *Oncologist*. 2013;18(1):19-24. doi: 10.1634/theoncologist.2012-0234. Epub 2013 Jan 8.

Yurkovitch M, Wong A, Lam JM. Solitary congenital self-healing Langerhans cell histiocytosis: a benign variant of Langerhans cell histiocytosis? *Dermatol Online J*. 2013 Jan 15;19(1):3.

In: Rare Diseases
Editors: Giorgio Di Giovanni and Pietro Marcoz
ISBN: 978-1-62948-525-6

Chapter V

Nail-Patella Syndrome

Sertac Cimen, Sanem Guler, Ryan Kelly, Frank MacDonald and Michele Molinari*
Department of Surgery, Dalhousie
University, Halifax, Nova Scotia, Canada

Abstract

Nail-patella syndrome (NPS) is an autosomal dominant disorder reported in 1/50000 individuals [1]. It has been mapped to the long arm of chromosome 9 (9q34) with mutations in LMX1B gene. Diagnosis is usually based on clinical findings. Cardinal anomalies of NPS are dysplasia of the nails, hypoplasia or absence of the patellae, presence of iliac horns and elbow abnormalities. Additionally some patients develop glomerulopathy and primary open angle glaucoma (POAG) along with other anomalies. Progression to renal failure occurs in about 10% of NPS patients requiring either dialysis or kidney transplantation.

Abbreviations

NPS	Nail-patella syndrome
HOOD	Hereditary onycho-osteodysplasia
DIP	Distal interphalangeal
PIP	Proximal interphalangeal
GBM	Glomerular basement membrane
POAG	Primary open angle glaucoma
ESRD	End stage renal disease
PAN	Polyarteritis Nodosa

* Corresponding author: Michele Molinari, 1276 South Park Street, Office 6-302 Victoria Building. E-mail: Michele.molinari@cdha.nshealth.ca; Fax: +1 902 473 7639.

BMD	Bone mineral density
MDD	Major depressive disorder
ADHD	Attention deficit hyperactivity disorder
PTLAH	Patella aplasia-hypoplasia
DOOR	Deafness-Onychoosteodystrophy-mental retardation
FISH	Fluorescence in Situ Hybridization
MRI	Magnetic Resonance Imaging
DEXA	Dual energy x-ray absorptiometry

Introduction

Nail-patella syndrome (NPS) is also known as Fong's Disease, Hereditary onycho-osteodysplasia (HOOD), Österreicher-Turner syndrome or Turner-Keiser syndrome [1, 2]. It is a rare hereditary autosomal dominant disorder reported in 1/50.000 live births and it has been described for the first time by Chatelaine in 1820 [1, 2]. The initial reports regarding the family cluster of the disease were published by Little in 1897, by Wrede in 1909 and by Beals and Eckhardt in 1969 [3, 4]. NPS is caused by heterozygous loss-of-function mutations of the LMX1B (LIM homeobox transcription factor 1-beta) gene which is located on the long arm of chromosome 9 (9q34) and linked to the ABO blood group locus [5-7]. LMX1B gene encodes LMX1B (NPS protein), a member of the LIM (Lin-1, Isl-1 and Mec-3)-homedomain family of transcription factors [8, 9]. It contains two motifs (LIM-A and LIM-B domain) and a homeodomain [5]. To date at least 142 LMX1B mutations have been identified [5]. These include missense/nonsense mutations and abnormal splicing mutations [5]. LMX1B is required for dorso-ventral patterning of the limb, differentiation of dopaminergic neurons, serotonergic neurons and podocytes, normal morphogenesis of the glomerular basement membrane (GBM) as well as anterior segment of the eye [5, 8].

Therefore patients afflicted by NPS show multi-organ involvement. Although it is a highly penetrant hereditary disorder, it shows marked inter- and intrafamilial phenotypic variability [5]. Extensive mutation analysis of different NPS families failed to demonstrate any genotype-phenotype correlation [5]. Since findings and manifestations are extremely variable, it is common that patients with NPS are undiagnosed even when they have a strong family history [10].

Clinical Diagnosis

NPS is characterized by a tetrad of 'cardinal anomalies' and potential 'associated anomalies' with involvement of numerous organs and body sites (Table 1).

Cardinal Anomalies

Cardinal anomalies include changes involving the nails, knees, elbows and iliac horns [10]. Diagnosis is based on these cardinal anomalies.

1. Nail Findings

Changes in the nails represent the most constant clinical features of patients with NPS [5]. Approximately 98% of the patients have nail findings including dystrophy, hypoplasia or aplasia [10]. Discoloration, cracking, spooning, thinning or thickening of the nails together with pits, longitudinal or horizontal ridges or clefts and triangle-shaped lunulae are the most common changes [5, 11]. Triangular lunulae on the thumbs are highly predictive for NPS so that some authors believe that they are pathognomonic [9, 12]. These changes may be seen at birth or may develop afterwards [10]. They are usually bilateral and more dominant in the hands, particularly in the thumbs [10]. Severity decreases toward the little finger [10]. When toenails are affected, little toenails are most commonly involved [10]. Flexion capacities of the distal interphalangeal (DIP) joints are usually reduced with consequential loss of the creases in the overlying skin [10]. This finding is most prominent in the index fingers even in patients with normal nails [9]. Proximal interphalangeal (PIP) joints may hyperextend whenever DIP joints are flexed resulting in 'swan-neck' deformity and clinodactyly (curving of the fifth finger towards to fourth finger) [10].

2. Knee Findings

Knee anomalies are usually bilateral [10]. Patellar bones are small and dysplastic or absent [10] (Figure 1). Probably due to the abnormal development of the vastus medialis muscle, which contributes to correct tracking of the patella, subluxation or dislocation of the patellar bone is common [10].

Table 1. Summary of the most common characteristic anomalies of patients affected by nail-patella syndrome

References	Anomaly	Details	Frequency of presentation
[2, 5, 9]	Nail	Absence, hypoplasia or dystrophia	95%- 100%
[2]	Nail	Triangular lunulae	88%
[2, 5, 9]	Knee	Absent or hypoplastic patella	74%- 92%
[2]	Elbow	Dysplasia of the radial head, hypoplasia of the medial epicondyle	70%
[5]	Elbow	Elbow contracture	40%
[9]	Elbow	Dysplasia of the radial head, hypoplasia of the medial epicondyle	92%
[2, 5, 9]	Iliac bones	Iliac horns	53%-80%
[2, 5]	Kidneys	NPS nephropathy	26%-70%
[2, 5]	Kidneys	End stage renal disease	5%-10%
[2, 27, 28]	Eyes	Primary open angle glaucoma	10%-30%
[2]	Feet	Pes planus	64%
[2]	Chest wall	Pectus excavatum	36%
[2]	Spinal column	Increased lumbar lordosis	47%
[2]	Circulatory system	Raynaud's phenomenon	55%
[2]	Nervous system	Peripheral neurological symptoms	25%
[2]	Gastrointestinal system	Constipation	18%
[2]	Teeth	Weak, crumbling teeth with thin enamel	23%

Up to 74% of patients display recurrent subluxation or dislocation of the patellae, leading to chronic pain and disruption of the extensor mechanism of the knee, often exacerbated by exercise [2, 10]. Prominent medial femoral condyles and tibial tuberosities together with hypoplastic lateral femoral condyles and patella give a flattened appearance to the knee [10]. When present, the patella is frequently tripartite or polygonal [11]. Other potential findings are genu valgum (inward slant of the knee when the legs are straightened), genu recurvatum (backward-bending knee), genu varum (outward bowing of the leg), osteochondritis dissecans (a joint condition in which a piece of cartilage along with a thin layer of the bone beneath it comes loose from the end of the bone) and hypoplasia or absence of anterior cruciate ligaments [2]. Early degenerative arthritis is common [10]. Hamstring muscles (semitendinosus, semimembranosus and biceps femoris muscles which make up the borders of the space behind the knee) may be tight and cause flexion contractures in the knees [10]. A midline synovial septum completely subdividing the knee joint into medial and lateral compartments has recently been reported as a potential arthroscopic finding [13]. Recurrence of this septum after surgical resection has also been described [13]. Patients with patellar involvement usually have symptoms including inability to straighten the knee joints, chronic pain, clicking and locking of the knees [10].

3. Iliac Horns

Iliac horns are bilateral conical exostoses (bony processes) that project posterolaterally from the central part of the iliac bones [10] (Figure 2). Iliac horns were first described by Turner in 1933 as 'iliac crest flaring with prominent anterior superior spines' [3]. In 1946, Fong applied the term 'iliac horns' to the list of abnormalities associated with NPS [14].

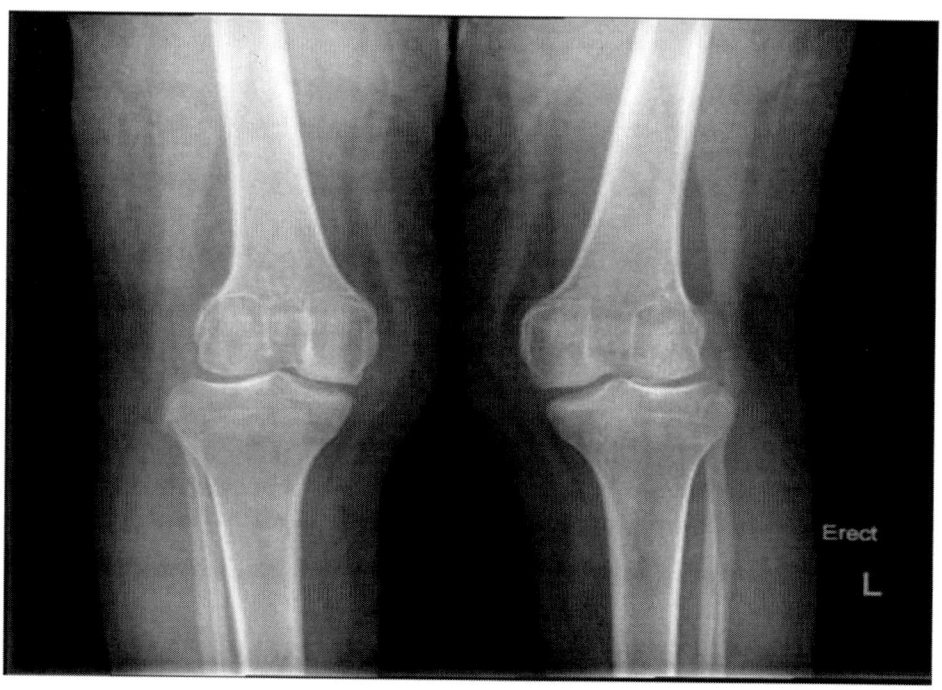

Figure 1. Example of a bilateral knee X-ray of a patient affected by nail-patella syndrome. The patellae are absent and there are characteristic valgus knee joints.

Today, iliac horns are considered pathognomonic for NPS [10]. They can be detected in up to 70% of the patients [10]. Iliac horns may be visible, palpable in the substance of glutei or impalpable depending on their size [15]. They are asymptomatic even when palpable [10].

4. Elbow Findings

Elbow involvement is usually bilateral and present in almost 70% of the patients [10]. Elbow findings include dysplasia of the radial head, hypoplasia of the lateral epicondyle and capitellum and prominence of the medial epicondyles [10]. These changes, which are similar to the changes in the knees can be responsible for dislocations of the elbow joint [10]. Cubitus valgus (lateral angling of the forearm to a greater degree than normal (>29°) in full extension) and antecubital pterygia (antecubital webbing with posterior subluxation of the radial head and maldevelopment of radioulnar joint) may also be associated [10].

Associated Anomalies

There are many other potential associated anomalies that may be seen in NPS patients by involvement of other organs such as kidneys, eyes, ankles, feet, spinal column, chest wall, teeth, gastrointestinal, neurologic and circulatory systems:

1. Renal Involvement

Renal impairment was initially described by Hawkins and Smith in 1950 with patients presenting with clinical features of chronic glomerulonephritis [16]. Thirty to fifty percent of NPS patients have renal involvement [2].

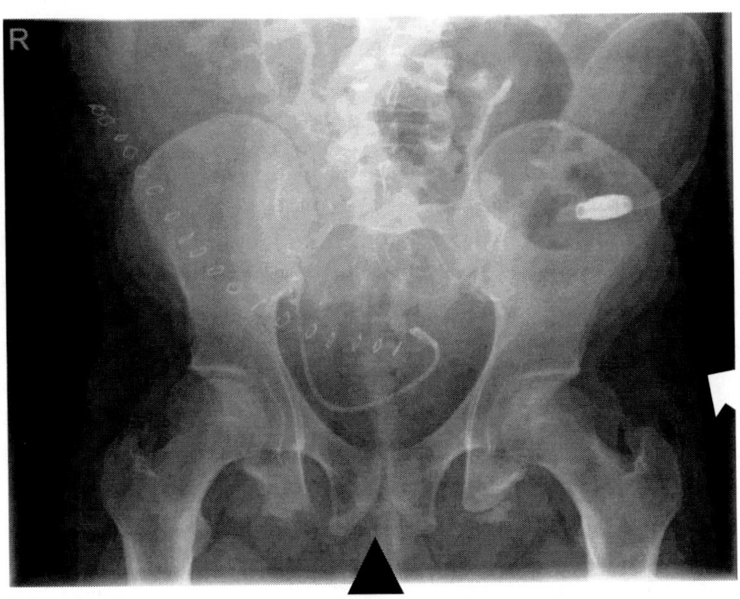

Figure 2. Abdominal X-ray of a patient with nail-patella syndrome who underwent renal transplantation in the right iliac fossa. The characteristic iliac horn is more visible on the left iliac crest (white arrow). A double J ureteral stent inserted during renal transplantation is visible in the right iliac fossa (black arrow).

Although common in adults, it has also been reported in children and infants [10, 17]. The mean age at detection is 21.7 years (range: 1-51) [2]. It was found to be significantly more frequent in females than males [5, 18]. Positive family history of nephropathy and presence of radial head hypoplasia are associated with an increased risk of developing renal disease with edema, hypertension and proteinuria [5, 18]. LMX1B (NPS protein) plays an important role in morphogenesis and function of GBM and podocytes [2]. It is also required for regulation of collagen type IV expression [19]. Accordingly, the most common renal pathologic findings of NPS are focal or diffuse thickening of the GBM with patchy electron-lucent areas ('moth-eaten' appearance), podocyte foot process effacement and irregular deposition of bundles of fibrillar collagen (type 3 collagen) within the GBM and the mesangial matrix [5]. However, the severity of these changes does not correlate well with the severity of proteinuria and the degree of renal impairment [5]. One of the characteristics of NPS is that, there are no specific light microscopy or immunofluorescence features [20]. The earliest sign of renal involvement of NPS is proteinuria [5, 10]. Proteinuria may present at any time from birth onwards and may be intermittent and associated with hematuria [10]. Sixty percent of patients present with non-nephrotic proteinuria. Patients with mutations located in the homeodomain have significantly higher risk for proteinuria than subjects carrying mutations in the LIM domains [18, 20]. Proteinuria may remain asymptomatic, remit spontaneously or may progress to nephrotic syndrome or nephritis [10, 21]. Two patterns of nephropathy can be distinguished [22]. Most of the patients manifest solely an accelerated age-related loss of filtration function in comparison to the unaffected individuals [22]. Proteinuria does not seem to be progressive and progression to symptomatic kidney failure is very uncommon [22]. On the other hand, 5-10% of patients with NPS develop nephrotic-range proteinuria in infancy, childhood or early adulthood and progress to end stage renal disease (ESRD) [22]. Factors responsible for this progression have not been identified yet [5]. Since progression to ESRD occurs in about 10% of NPS patients, renal impairment is considered as one of the major prognostic factors of NPS [2, 5]. Renal impairment may occur for the first time or may be exacerbated during pregnancy and the incidence of pre-eclampsia was found to be significantly higher (29%) in NPS when compared to the general population (2-5%) [10, 20]. Minimal change disease, Goodpasture's Syndrome, IgA nephropathy, hemolytic uremic syndrome, membranous nephropathy, polyarteritis nodosa (PAN)-type vasculitis have been reported as incidental clinical entities in the setting of NPS [3, 21, 23-26].

2. Ocular Involvement

NPS patients are afflicted by primary open-angle glaucoma (POAG) more often and at younger ages than the general population [2, 27]. Even so, POAG usually develops during adulthood and requires early diagnosis and treatment to avoid asymptomatic visual field loss and eventual blindness [28]. Although not considered as pathognomonic, pigmentary changes in the iris leading to a clover-shaped zone of darker pigmentation (Lester's sign) around the centre of the iris are frequently seen in NPS [10]. Ocular hypertension, normal-tension and congenital glaucoma are also associated with NPS [27]. Keratoconus (degenerative disorder of the eye in which structural changes within the cornea cause it to thin and change to a more conical shape than its normal gradual curve), microcornea, microphakia (abnormal smallness of the lens), hyperpigmentation of pupillary margins, cataracts and ptosis can be detected as well [15]. Ectopic cilia have been reported recently as a rare coexisting entity [29].

3. Ankle and Feet Involvement

Achilles tendons of NPS patients are usually tight and this feature may lead to talipes equinovarus (club foot; foot rotated internally at the ankle) and toe-walking [10].

Additionally, hyperdorsiflexion of the foot, talipes equinovalgus (plantar-flexed, everted and abducted foot due to combination of talipes equines and talipes valgus), calcaneovalgus (dorsiflexed, everted and abducted foot due to combination of talipes calcaneus and talipes valgus), calcaneovarus (dorsiflexed, inverted and adducted foot due to combination of talipes calcaneus and talipes varus) and pes planus (lowering of the longitudinal arch) can be encountered in NPS patients [10].

4. Spinal Column Involvement

Spondylolysis (defect in the pars interarticularis of the vertebral arch), spondylolisthesis (anterior or posterior displacement of a vertebra), spina bifida occulta, mild scoliosis (lateral curve in the spine) and increased lumbar lordosis (increased inward curving of the lumbar spine) can be seen in NPS patients [2, 10]. Approximately half of the patients complain about back pain [10].

5. Chest Involvement

Pectus excavatum (inward sinking of the sternum) can be associated with NPS [10]. Additionally hypoplasia of the scapulae and the first ribs, scapular winging and clavicular horn (conical spine like projection in the lateral aspect of the clavicle) may be present [11, 15].

6. Teeth Involvement

Weak, easily-disintegrating teeth with thin dental enamel are signs of dental involvement [10].

7. Gastrointestinal Involvement

Constipation or irritable bowel syndrome are indicators of gastrointestinal involvement [10].

8. Neurological Involvement

Reduced pain and temperature sensation, intermittent numbness, tingling and burning sensations (paresthesia) in hands and feet are signs and symptoms exhibited by many NPS patients [10, 30]. The paresthesia is usually in a glove and stocking pattern [10, 30]. These problems may arise from the orthopedic changes associated with the disease which can cause potential neurological compromise [10, 30]. Approximately 6% of the patients have epilepsy [2].

9. Circulatory System (Vasomotor) Involvement

Vasomotor problems leading to poor peripheral circulation, cold hands and feet and Raynaud's phenomenon are quite common [10].

10. Other Features

Approximately 8-20% of the patients are afflicted by either osteoporosis or low bone mineral density (BMD) [10]. Hence, they have increased rate of bone fractures particularly before puberty [31]. Patients usually have lean body habitus, difficulty in gaining weight and decreased muscle mass although they have sufficient protein intake [10].

Impaired hearing, tilted uterus (retroverted uterus, tipped uterus), hypothyroidism, mental retardation, thyrotoxicosis, major depressive disorder (MDD), attention deficit hyperactivity disorder (ADHD), short stature, cleft lip and palate, OEIS complex (Omphalocele-extrophy-imperforate anus-spinal defects complex) can be rarely associated with NPS [11, 15, 32-34]. Haras et al. reported an NPS patient who had thyrotoxicosis as an associated finding [33]. However, they considered it as an incidental, unrelated clinical feature. They investigated the skeletal integrity and BMD of their patient further given that both thyrotoxicosis and NPS are risk factors for reduced BMD or osteoporosis.

Lopez-Arvizu et al. stated that NPS patients had increased rate of MDD and ADHD and ascribed this finding to mesencephalic dopaminergic neurologic pathway abnormalities that are a consequence of LMX1B loss of function [34]. Haddad and coworkers reported that 'short stature' might be the presenting symptom of the NPS patients [11].

Differential Diagnosis

Small patella syndrome, Patella aplasia-hypoplasia (PTLAH), Senior Syndrome, Rapadilino Syndrome, Coffin-Siris Syndrome, Trisomy 8 mosaicism (T8M), DOOR syndrome, genitopatellar syndrome, Meier-Gorlin Syndrome and familial recurrent dislocation of the patella syndrome are the syndromes that enter the differential diagnosis of NPS [10, 35-45].

Similarities and differences among these syndromes and NPS are presented in Table 2. It is important to note that renal manifestations of an NPS patient may be due to other co-incidental clinical entities. As mentioned above, minimal change disease, Goodpasture's Syndrome, IgA nephropathy, hemolytic uremic syndrome, membranous nephropathy and polyarteritis nodosa (PAN)-type vasculitis have been reported in NPS patients with or without histopathological evidence of NPS nephropathy [3, 21, 23-26].

Hence, renal biopsy must be performed and the specific histopathological renal biopsy findings of NPS nephropathy must be confirmed before ascribing the renal manifestations of the NPS patient to NPS nephropathy. This approach will also help in diagnosing these clinical entities-which can be present in the absence of NPS nephropathy- on time, before causing irreversible damage.

The most important differential diagnosis of the NPS nephropathy is collagenofibrotic glomerulopathy (collagen type III glomerulopathy) [46]. They are both characterized by pathological accumulation of collagen type III in glomeruli; in GBM, mesangium and capillary walls [17, 46, 47].

However, it must be considered that glomerular involvement in NPS invariably presents in patients with the multiorgan disorder with orthopedic manifestations [46].

Table 2. Comparison of the findings of NPS with other syndromes that enter its differential diagnosis

References	Syndrome	Similarities	Differences
[10, 35]	Small patella syndrome	Small or absent patellae, recurrent patellar dislocation, pelvic anomalies	No nail and elbow changes, no renal or ocular involvement, infra-acetabular 'axe-cut' notch, ischial hypoplasia
[10, 36]	Patella aplasia-hypoplasia	Patellar aplasia or hypoplasia	No nail and elbow changes, no renal or ocular involvement
[10, 37, 38]	Familial recurrent dislocation of patella	Recurrent patellar dislocation, genu valgum	Bilateral short fourth and fifth metatarsi, no nail and elbow changes, no renal or ocular involvement
[10, 39]	Meier-Gorlin syndrome	Absent patellae, recurrent radial head dislocation	Markedly short stature, characteristic facial appearance
[10, 40]	Genitopatellar syndrome	Absent patellae, club foot	Facial dysmorphism, genital anomalies, microcephaly, hypoplasia of the ischia and iliac bones
[10, 41]	DOOR syndrome	Absent or hypoplastic nails	Long and/or triphalangeal thumbs, long big toes, short fingers, structural abnormalities of the urinary tract, optic atrophy, Dandy-Walker malformation, ptosis, deafness, mental retardation
[10, 42, 43]	Trisomy 8 mosaicism	Absent or hypoplastic patellae, nail abnormalities, limited supination capacity of the elbow joint	Facial dysmorphism, camptodactyly, deep plantar creases
[10, 44]	Coffin-Siris syndrome	Recurrent elbow dislocation, absence or hypoplasia of nails and patellae	Facial dysmorphism, nail hypoplasia dominant in little finger nails
[10]	Rapadilino syndrome	Hypoplastic or absent patellae, joint dislocations, radial defects	Absent or hypoplastic thumbs and radii, facial dysmorphism
[10, 45]	Senior syndrome	Small nails	Characteristic facial appearance (broad nose, flat malar area, large mouth, pointed chin)

DOOR syndrome (Deafness, Onychdystrophy, Osteodistrophy and Mental Retardation).

Genetic Diagnosis

Although genetic tests are not indispensable for the diagnosis of NPS in individuals presenting with the classical clinical features of the disease, there are some occasions that warrant genetic testing [10]:

- Patients with atypical phenotype or patients with signs and symptoms beyond the typical NPS phenotype
- Failure in the clinical/histopathological differential diagnosis process
- Prenatal/pre-implantation diagnosis in at-risk pregnancies

The sole gene, mutation of which is known to cause NPS is LMX1B [10]. Approximately 88% of NPS patients have an affected parent [10]. However, inheritance of a mutated allele from an unaffected parent with somatic mosaicism has also been reported [48]. On the other hand, 12% of the affected patients have a *de novo* mutation [48]. Both sexes are affected in equal numbers [11]. Cytogenetic testing as well as molecular genetic testing is available for demonstrating the disrupted gene in NPS patients [10]. Cytogenetic testing can demonstrate the potential chromosomal translocations related to NPS nevertheless it represents a very uncommon mechanism for LMX1B mutation [10]. Sequence analysis, deletion/duplication analysis and Fluorescence in Situ Hybridization (FISH) are the main methods for molecular genetic testing [10]. Sequence analysis can detect 85% of the LMX1B mutations leading to NPS [10]. Mutations in sequence variants (exons 2 through 6) revealed by sequence analysis is related to NPS [10]. Another molecular genetic testing method is deletion-duplication testing and it can detect approximately 5% of the mutations [10]. Exonic or whole-gene deletions can be detected by this method in relation to NPS [10]. FISH analysis can reveal the large deletions in the target gene [10]. Being an autosomal dominant disorder, the probability of having an affected child is 50% per pregnancy hence genetic counseling must be considered [15]. Prenatal diagnosis for at-risk pregnancies is possible if the disease causing mutation is identified in the family [10]. It is performed by analysis of the DNA extracted from fetal cells obtained by either amniocentesis at 15-18 weeks or chorionic villous sampling at 10-12 weeks of pregnancy [10]. However, it must be considered that these tests can determine whether or not the fetus has inherited the disease-causing mutation, but they cannot predict the phenotype, namely 'severity of the clinical manifestations' [10]. Preimplantation genetic diagnosis is also available for families in which the relevant mutation has been identified [10].

Management after Initial Diagnosis

Diagnosis of NPS warrants further investigative work-up to assess the extent of the disease and possible dysfunction of the other organs [10].

Urinalysis should be used to assess presence of proteinuria and urine albumin-creatinine ratio and blood pressure measurements must be obtained to screen for renal insufficiency [10].

Patients must be referred to a nephrologist if this preliminary investigation raises any suspicion [10]. Renal biopsy is crucial for diagnosis of NPS nephropathy and exclusion or diagnosis of other potential co-incidental renal diseases [5, 20, 21].

Eye examination is important as the presence of POAG is a significant risk for vision impairment and blindness [5]. Abnormal or absent red reflex is an alarming sign for immediate referral to an ophthalmologist [10]. Patients must have intra-ocular pressure assessment during childhood as well as assessment of visual fields and optic disc.

Clues regarding orthopedic problems and potential gastrointestinal, neurological, vasomotor and dental involvement can be obtained during history taking and physical examination: Dislocation in the knee and/or elbow joint, knee pain, clicking and locking in the knees, back pain, bone fractures, constipation or alternating bouts of constipation and diarrhea with flatulence, numbness, tingling and burning sensations in hands and feet, seizures, color changes in fingers especially when exposed to cold and crumbling teeth are very important symptoms and findings.

Magnetic Resonance Imaging (MRI) and dual energy x-ray absorptiometry (DEXA) are very important diagnostic tools for radiologic assessment of the bone and soft tissue abnormalities and evaluation of the osteoporosis and bone fracture risk [10].

Treatment and Surveillance

Orthopedic Manifestations

Although most of the orthopedic problems associated with NPS are 'congenital' rather than acquired, some of them bear the potential to cause 'acquired' deformities (e.g., 'swan-neck' deformity, clinodactyly, flexion contractures in the knees) if remains untreated [10]. Hence, one of the most important goals of the treatment regarding orthopedic manifestations of NPS is prevention of the acquired problems. On the other hand, treatment may be needed solely for 'symptomatic' relief. Thus, a variety of therapeutic methods including analgesics, physical therapy and rehabilitation, splinting, bracing and surgery can be involved in treatment of the orthopedic problems [10]. Chronic use of non-steroid anti-inflammatory drugs must be avoided because of their potential impact on kidney function [10].

Renal Manifestations

Surveillance with annual measurement of blood pressure, urinalysis and urine albumin-creatinine ratio is crucial for early diagnosis of renal impairment and referral to nephrologist on time [10]. Nephrotic syndrome due to NPS nephropathy is resistant to therapy with corticosteroids [21]. However, it has been reported that antiproteinuric treatment with combination of angiotensin converting enzyme inhibitor and angiotensin receptor blocker can provide complete remission in infantile nephrotic syndrome secondary to NPS [17]. On the other hand, nephrotic syndrome diagnosed as an incidental comorbidity in the setting of NPS without NPS nephropathy may respond to steroid treatment similar to the general population [21].

Hypertensive NPS patients are treated as in the general population and kidney transplantation has been used to treat patients who progressed to end-stage renal failure [49]. In this case, results are usually favorable and there is no risk for post-transplant recurrence [10, 15].

Chan et al. performed live-related kidney transplantation in a recipient with NPS [49]. Graft biopsy done 18 months post-transplantation revealed normal GBM by electron microscopy [49]. Interestingly, this patient's previously dystrophic index finger nails had re-grown hence the authors suggested that the transplanted donor kidney might be replenishing the deficient factor (i.e., NPS protein) [49]. To the best of our knowledge, re-growth of the dystrophic nails or any improvement in the other cardinal findings of the syndrome post-transplant has not been observed by other authors.

Vega et al. reported a kidney transplantation from a cadaveric donor with NPS to a recipient with ESRD due to chronic glomerulonephritis [50]. The authors did not know that the donor had NPS [50]. They diagnosed NPS nephropathy by graft biopsy performed 8 days after the transplantation with the indication of suspicion of acute rejection [50]. After a satisfactory follow-up period of 11 years, these authors suggested that NPS did not have significant influence on the survival of the graft [50]. They concluded that kidneys from donors afflicted with NPS could be used for transplantation, unless there is clinically obvious renal impairment [50].

Ocular Manifestations

Screening for glaucoma starting from the time that the child is compliant with the relevant ocular examination is crucial [10]. Treatment is as in the general population for patients with intraocular hypertension or glaucoma [10].

Other Manifestations

Other manifestations of NPS are all treated as in the general population. Dental examination every 6 months and periodic DEXA scanning are indicated due to potential dental involvement and risk of osteoporosis or low BMD [10]. Early diagnosis of osteoporosis or low BMD is important since functional outcome after bone fractures may be inferior to the general population [51].

References

[1] Mimiwati, Z., Mackey, D. A., Craig, J. E., et al.: Nail-patella syndrome and its association with glaucoma: a review of eight families. *Br. J. Ophthalmol.* 2006;90: 1505-9.

[2] Sweeney, E., Fryer, A., Mountford, R., Green, A., McIntosh, I.: Nail patella syndrome: a review of the phenotype aided by developmental biology. *J. Med. Genet.* 2003;40: 153-62.

[3] Croock, A. D., Bashar Kahaleh, M., Powers, J. M.: Vasculitis and renal disease in nail-patella syndrome: case report and literature review. *Ann. Rheum. Dis.* 1987;46:562-5.

[4] Beals, R. K., Eckhardt, A. L.: Hereditary onycho-osteodysplasia (Nail-Patella syndrome). A report of nine kindreds. *J. Bone Joint Surg. Am.* 1969;51:505-16.

[5] Lee, B. H., Cho, T. J., Choi, H. J., et al.: Clinico-genetic study of nail-patella syndrome. *J. Korean Med. Sci.* 2009;24 Suppl.: S82-6.

[6] Chatterjee, M., Chatterjee, C.: Nail-patella syndrome--a preliminary study for genetic linkage with ABO blood group. *J. Indian Med. Assoc.* 2010;108:747-9.

[7] Dreyer, S. D., Zhou, G., Baldini, A., et al.: Mutations in LMX1B cause abnormal skeletal patterning and renal dysplasia in nail patella syndrome. *Nat. Genet.* 1998;19: 47-50.

[8] Dai, J. X., Johnson, R. L., Ding, Y. Q.: Manifold functions of the Nail-Patella Syndrome gene Lmx1b in vertebrate development. *Dev. Growth Differ.* 2009;51:241-50.

[9] Bongers, E. M., Gubler, M. C., Knoers, N. V.: Nail-patella syndrome. Overview on clinical and molecular findings. *Pediatr. Nephrol.* 2002;17:703-12.

[10] Sweeney, E., Hoover-Fong, J. E., McIntosh, I.: *Nail-Patella Syndrome*. 1993.

[11] Haddad, S., Ghedira-Besbes, L., Bouafsoun, C., et al.: Nail-patella syndrome associated with short stature: a case series. *Case Rep. Med.* 2010;2010.

[12] Richert, B., Andre, J.: Nail disorders in children: diagnosis and management. *Am. J. Clin. Dermatol.* 2011;12:101-12.

[13] Heckman, D. S., McCoy, A. J., Spritzer, C. E., Garrett, W. E.: Intercondylar Synovial Septum in Two Patients with Nail-Patella Syndrome. *J. Knee Surg.* 2012.

[14] Fong, E. E.: Iliac horns (symmetrical bilateral central posterior iliac processes). *Radiology* 1946;47:517.

[15] Senguttuvan, N. B., Sivaraman, A., Kandasamy, D., Marimuthu, K.: Nail patella syndrome: a rare cause of renal failure in a young adult. *Pan. Afr. Med. J.* 2011;9:31.

[16] Hawkins, C. F., Smith, O. E.: Renal dysplasia in a family with multiple hereditary abnormalities including iliac horns. *Lancet* 1950;1:803-8.

[17] Proesmans, W., Van Dyck, M., Devriendt, K.: Nail-patella syndrome, infantile nephrotic syndrome: complete remission with antiproteinuric treatment. *Nephrol. Dial. Transplant* 2009;24:1335-8.

[18] Bongers, E. M., Huysmans, F. T., Levtchenko, E., et al.: Genotype-phenotype studies in nail-patella syndrome show that LMX1B mutation location is involved in the risk of developing nephropathy. *Eur. J. Hum. Genet.* 2005;13:935-46.

[19] Bongers, E. M., Knoers, N. V.: [From gene to disease; the nail-patella syndrome and the LMX1B gene]. *Ned Tijdschr Geneeskd* 2003;147:67-9.

[20] Sood, P., Rojas, M. C., Talor, Z.: Renal involvement in nail-patella syndrome: report of three cases. *Int. Urol. Nephrol.* 2010;42:499-502.

[21] Hari, P., Mantan, M., Dinda, A., Hari, S., Bagga, A.: Steroid-responsive nephrotic syndrome in a patient with nail-patella syndrome. *Pediatr. Nephrol.* 2006;21:1197-9.

[22] Lemley, K. V.: Kidney disease in nail-patella syndrome. *Pediatr. Nephrol.* 2009;24: 2345-54.

[23] Curtis, J. J., Bhathena, D., Leach, R. P., Galla, J. H., Lucas, B. A., Luke, R. G.: Goodpasture's syndrome in a patient with the Nail-Patella syndrome. *Am. J. Med.* 1976; 61:401-6.

[24] Gao, X., Miyai, T., Tahara, T., et al.: IgA nephropathy associated with Nail-Patella syndrome in a 7-year-old girl. *Pediatr. Int.* 2001;43:434-6.

[25] Robson, W. L., Leung, A. K.: Diarrhea-associated hemolytic-uremic syndrome in a child with nail-patella syndrome. *South Med. J.* 1995;88:780-1.

[26] Mackay, I. G., Doig, A., Thomson, D.: Membranous nephropathy in a patient with nail-patella syndrome nephropathy. *Scott. Med. J.* 1985;30:47-9.

[27] Lichter, P. R., Richards, J. E., Downs, C. A., Stringham, H. M., Boehnke, M., Farley, F. A.: Cosegregation of open-angle glaucoma and the nail-patella syndrome. *Am. J. Ophthalmol.* 1997;124:506-15.

[28] Park, S., Jamshidi, Y., Vaideanu, D., Bitner-Glindzicz, M., Fraser, S., Sowden, J. C.: Genetic risk for primary open-angle glaucoma determined by LMX1B haplotypes. *Invest. Ophthalmol. Vis. Sci.* 2009;50:1522-30.

[29] Edmunds, M. R., Kipioti, A., Colloby, P. S., Reuser, T. T.: A case of ectopic cilia in nail-patella syndrome. *Int. Ophthalmol.* 2012;32:289-92.

[30] Dunston, J. A., Reimschisel, T., Ding, Y. Q., et al.: A neurological phenotype in nail patella syndrome (NPS) patients illuminated by studies of murine Lmx1b expression. *Eur. J. Hum. Genet.* 2005;13:330-5.

[31] Towers, A. L., Clay, C. A., Sereika, S. M., McIntosh, I., Greenspan, S. L.: Skeletal integrity in patients with nail patella syndrome. *J. Clin. Endocrinol. Metab.* 2005;90: 1961-5.

[32] Zen, P. R., Rosa, R. F., Graziadio, C., da Silva, A. P., Paskulin, G. A.: Omphalocele-exstrophy-imperforate anus-spinal defects (OEIS) complex in a child with nail-patella syndrome. *Pediatr. Int.* 2010;52:847-8.

[33] Haras, B., Vulpoi, F., Onose, G.: A case of nail-patella syndrome associated with thyrotoxicosis. *J. Med. Life* 2012;5:126-9.

[34] Lopez-Arvizu, C., Sparrow, E. P., Strube, M. J., et al.: Increased symptoms of attention deficit hyperactivity disorder and major depressive disorder symptoms in Nail-patella syndrome: potential association with LMX1B loss-of-function. *Am. J. Med. Genet. B Neuropsychiatr. Genet.* 2011;156B:59-66.

[35] Bongers, E. M., Duijf, P. H., van Beersum, S. E., et al.: Mutations in the human TBX4 gene cause small patella syndrome. *Am. J. Hum. Genet.* 2004;74:1239-48.

[36] Mangino, M., Sanchez, O., Torrente, I., et al.: Localization of a gene for familial patella aplasia-hypoplasia (PTLAH) to chromosome 17q21-22. *Am. J. Hum. Genet.* 1999;65: 441-7.

[37] Miller, G. F.: Familial recurrent dislocation of the patella. *J. Bone Joint Surg. Br.* 1978; 60-B:203-4.

[38] Borochowitz, Z., Soudry, M., Mendes, D. G.: Familial recurrent dislocation of patella with autosomal dominant mode of inheritance. *Clin. Genet.* 1988;33:1-4.

[39] De Munnik, S. A., Otten, B. J., Schoots, J., et al.: Meier-Gorlin syndrome: growth and secondary sexual development of a microcephalic primordial dwarfism disorder. *Am. J. Med. Genet.* A 2012;158A:2733-42.

[40] To, M., Negandhi, R., Cheung, K., Cheung, W. Y., Chow, W.: Genitopatellar syndrome: a case report of a rare entity with 11 years of follow-up. *J. Pediatr. Orthop. B* 2013;22:333-8.

[41] James, A. W., Miranda, S. G., Culver, K., Hall, B. D., Golabi, M.: DOOR syndrome: clinical report, literature review and discussion of natural history. *Am. J. Med. Genet. A* 2007;143A:2821-31.

[42] Fineman, R. M., Ablow, R. C., Howard, R. O., Albright, J., Breg, W. R.: Trisomy 8 mosaicism syndrome. *Pediatrics* 1975;56:762-7.

[43] Agrawal, A., Agrawal, R.: Warkany syndrome: a rare case report. *Case Rep. Pediatr.* 2011;2011:437101.

[44] Carey, J. C., Hall, B. D.: The Coffin-Siris syndrome: five new cases including two siblings. *Am. J. Dis. Child* 1978;132:667-71.

[45] Verloes, A., Bonneau, D., Guidi, O., et al.: Brachymorphism-onychodysplasia-dysphalangism syndrome. *J. Med. Genet.* 1993;30:158-61.

[46] Cohen, A. H.: Collagen Type III Glomerulopathies. *Adv. Chronic Kidney Dis.* 2012;19: 101-6.

[47] Salcedo, J. R.: An autosomal recessive disorder with glomerular basement membrane abnormalities similar to those seen in the nail patella syndrome: report of a kindred. *Am. J. Med. Genet.* 1984;19:579-84.

[48] Marini, M., Bocciardi, R., Gimelli, S., et al.: A spectrum of LMX1B mutations in Nail-Patella syndrome: new point mutations, deletion, and evidence of mosaicism in unaffected parents. *Genet. Med.* 2010;12:431-9.

[49] Chan, P. C., Chan, K. W., Cheng, I. K., Chan, M. K.: Living-related renal transplantation in a patient with nail-patella syndrome. *Nephron* 1988;50:164-6.

[50] Vega, F., Errasti, P., Pardo-Mindan, F. J.: Renal transplantation from a donor with a nail-patella syndrome. *Nephrol. Dial. Transplant* 1997;12:1742-4.

[51] Neill, S. C., Murphy, C. G., McElwain, J. P.: A hypoplastic patella fracture in nail patella syndrome: a case report. *J. Med. Case Rep.* 2012;6:196.

In: Rare Diseases
Editors: Giorgio Di Giovanni and Pietro Marcoz
ISBN: 978-1-62948-525-6

Chapter VI

Cardiac Angiosarcoma

Angela Lamarca*
Medical Oncology Department,
The Christie NHS Foundation Trust,
Manchester, UK

Abstract

Quality literature for management of cardiac angiosarcoma is shortly supplied due to the low incidence and its poor prognosis. A multidisciplinary management of these tumours is radically important, offering surgery or even cardiac transplant for the few potentially resectable patients. Even after complete resection, early recurrence and distant spread are the rule. Chemotherapy would be the treatment of choice for those patients diagnosed with distant metastases (56-80%) and for those with distant relapse after surgery. Most of the chemotherapy schedules employed are those with known efficacy for other soft tissue sarcoma. Nevertheless there are important characteristics in the pathology of these tumours that might have impact in the systemic treatment. As it happened with the Kaposi sarcoma, cardiac angiosarcomas are derived from endothelial cells and angiogenesis seems to be an important and druggable target. The employment of drugs with known antiangiogenic treatment like the anti-VEGF monoclonal antibody (bevacizumab) or multi-kinase inhibitors such as sorafenib and sunitib have been tested.

Epidemiology, diagnosis and management of cardiac angiosarcomas will be reviewed, focusing in the available data for target therapies.

Keywords: Angiosarcoma, heart, cardiac angiosarcoma, treatment, chemotherapy, target therapies

* Corresponding autor: Angela Lamarca, Medical Oncology Department, The Christie NHS Foundation Trust, Manchester, UK. E-mail: angelalamarca@hotmail.com.

Introduction

Angiosarcoma, the Concept

Angiosarcomas are malignant tumors that arise from the endothelial lining of blood vessels. They are classified as a rare subtype of soft tissue sarcomas: in fact, they constitute less than 1% of all soft tissue sarcomas. Angiosarcomas arise more commonly from skin, breast, bone, liver, and spleen. The overall survival for this subtype of soft tissue sarcoma is poor, with 5-year overall survival rates of 24% to 31% [1, 2].

By histology, most cases of angiosarcoma show complex vessels lined by atypical endothelial cells and intratumoral hemorrhage [3]. Sometimes, the vascular differentiation is so subtle, that hematoxylin and eosin–stained sections and vascular immunohistochemical vascular markers (CD31 and CD34) may be required for its recognition. The presence of atypical vessels at the periphery and, when present, intratumoural hemorrhage are clues for the pathological diagnosis.

Cardiac Tumours: Epidemiology and Diagnosis

Even primary cardiac tumors are rare (0.0001 to 0.03% of all tumors), they represent an important group of cardiovascular disease due to the importance of an accurate diagnosis [4]. Almost 90% of primary cardiac tumours are benign, with nearly 80% of them representing myxomas. Other subtypes of bening primary cardiac tumours include papillary fibroelastomas (26%), fibromas (6%) and lipomas (4%). Only about 10% of primary cardiac tumours are malignant, of which more than 90% are sarcomas (the most common histological subtype is angiosarcoma) [5].

However, we might not forget that, secondary malignant heart tumours are, by far, much more frequent than the primary ones: between 30-1000 times more common. The most frequent underlying neoplasms with secondary cardiac metastases include: lung, breast, upper-gastrointestinal malignancies, renal, melanoma, lymphoma and leukaemia [6].

The clinical presentation of these cardiac masses is widely variable and usually determined by the location of the tumour rather than by its histologic subtype. Therefore, on the first hand, some tumours may be locally invasive, impairing myocardial contractility or causing valve dysfunction, and thus, presenting with heart failure, pulmonary embolism, fatal arrhythmias or pericardial effusion (with or without tamponade).

On the other hand, some patients may not present any cardiovascular symptoms and the diagnosis can be incidental. Finally, tumours of the aortic valve and left atrium present the highest embolic risk.

For the diagnosis of cardiac tumours, echocardiography is an ideal initial imaging modality (simple, non-invasive, widely available and low cost). The echocardiography is able to give information about the morphologic appearance, location and hemodynamic consequences of the tumour.

Further study with CT and MRI provide additional information, being useful for an accurate diagnosis, staging and treatment planning. Moreover, MRI can also provide information about vascularity and calcification [6].

Cardiac Angiosarcoma: What Do We Know?

Because of the low incidence and its poor prognosis, the scientific evidence for diagnosis and management is low, being mostly case reports and case series.

Most cardiac angiosarcomas are diagnosed between the third and fifth decade of life, with higher incidence in men than in women (ratio 2:1) [7]. Most of the primary heart angiosarcomas (90%) arise from right cavities. Presented symptoms at diagnosis depend on the grade of cardiac and pericardial invasion.

Therefore, potential symptoms at diagnosis may be: dyspnea, chest pain, hemoptysis, orthopnea and anorexia. Due to its aggressiveness and its location, pericardial effusion is frequently present and therefore, patients are usually diagnosed with cardiac tamponade, heart failure or right superior vena cava syndrome [4].

One of the more recent case series published estimated the median overall survival of patients with cardiac angiosarcoma at 13 months, while the overall survival for the subgroup of patients diagnosed with distant metastases was around 6 months [8].

Some studies analyzed potential prognostic factors: the involvement of the left heart compared to the involvement of the right heart, low number of mitotic cells and low presence of tumor necrosis in the tumour sample seemed to be related to a better prognostic [9]. Therefore, even the prognosis for patients with cardiac sarcomas is poor, according to some experts, histologic grading is useful in predicting outcome, and may be worth it [10].

As we discussed above, the first approach to the diagnosis of cardiac tumours is made by standard image techniques as echocardiography, CT or MRI. Performing a cardiac MRI when a cardiac angiosarcoma is suspected is usually worth it due to the information collected from those MRI sequences sensitive for hemorrhage (T1 weighted images). These sequences may show areas of hemorrhage (diffuse or nodular) with enhancement along vascular lakes after the administration of intravenous contrast (gadolinium-DTPA) [6].

However, the final diagnosis is obtained by pathologic examination of the primary lesion or a metastatic lesion [9]. Paradoxically, despite the frequent involvement of the pericardium, pericardial fluid cytology has low diagnostic sensitivity [11].

According to a series of 10 cardiac sarcomas analyzed, tumors are usually hemorrhagic, with variegated tan-brown solid areas and with mixed solid growth and anatomizing channels. Frequent mitoses and tumor necrosis are common, with high rate of Ki-67 expression and strong staining for CD31 and CD34 (see above) but negative for AE1/3, D2-40, human herpesvirus 8, and epidermal growth factor receptor [12].

Management of Primary Cardiac Angiosarcomas

To summarize, primary cardiac angiosarcoma is a rare but the most common malignant neoplasm of the heart in adults with very poor prognosis due to the high rate of distant metastases. The multidisciplinar management of these tumors is extremely important. In localized stages (without metastatic disease) surgery is the main curative option of treatment, while chemotherapy is the cornerstone of therapy for metastatic disease.

Localized Disease: Surgery, Adjuvant Therapy, Transplant

Those patients diagnosed in localized stages, without distant metastases, may benefit from a local treatment which is usually based on a surgical resection. However, due to the location of the primary tumour, the chances of a complete resection are very low. Some series have shown that having a complete resection is one of the most important prognostic related factors [7]. Selected patients with locally advanced tumours might benefit from a heart transplant even the benefit is not very well defined [13].

However, even after a complete resection, early recurrence and distant spread is the rule: the disease free survival is between 5 and 8 months after resection [4, 14]. In order to decrease the risk of relapse and distant metastases, adjuvant treatment has been employed in some case reports and case series.

- Slepicka et al. reported a case report of a primary cardiac angiosarcoma who was treated with surgical resection of the primary tumor, reconstruction of the right atrium and patch repair of the atrial septum [14]. After surgery, the patient underwent adjuvant radiation therapy to the atrial bed. Eight months later, the patient had distant metastases (bone and retroperitoneal lymph nodes), even no local relapse was shown.
- In 1998 a case series of 15 patients treated with adjuvant doxorubicin failed to show benefit due to the high rate of local recurrence [15]. The median relapse free survival was 10 months and 12 out of 15 patients had local relapse. In this study, other non-angiosarcoma primary cardiac sarcomas (9/15) were included. Having a complete resection was related with good prognosis, while the survival was also longer in those non-angiosarcoma tumours.
- In 2008 other case reported the benefit of neadjuvant treatment for a primary cardiac angiosarcoma of the right atrium with systemic metastases to the pericardium, superior vena cava, and lungs [16]. The patient received neoadjuvant and adjuvant chemotherapy with doxorubicin and complete surgical resection of the tumor with reconstruction of the right atrium using bovine pericardium.
- Overall, the actual evidence for adjuvant treatment with radiotherapy or chemotherapy is low and it is based on case reports rather than prospective studies. However, the available data show encouraging results. Prospective studies may be important for clarifying its benefit.

Metastatic Disease: Chemotherapy and Target Therapies

Between 56-80% of patients are diagnosed with metastatic disease [8, 15]. The most common metastatic sites are lung, bone and liver. Metastases in the central nervous system, intestine, spleen, adrenal glands, pleura, diaphragm, kidney, thyroid and skin have also been described [9]. All these patients will be managed with palliative treatment, looking for better quality of live a trying to increase the survival by controlling the tumour growth.

Even, as detailed above, some encouraging results have been published with aggressive and multimodal therapy combining radiotherapy, chemotherapy and surgery [16], palliative chemotherapy is the main treatment for patients with distant metastases.

For selected patients with symptoms related to the primary tumour, palliative surgery or radiotherapy may be beneficial [7, 9].

When radiotherapy to the primary tumour is planned, the potential toxicity of this treatment needs to be clarified: while the recommend radiotherapy dose for other location soft tissues sarcomas reaches the 70cGy, a dose higher than 40cGy is usually not tolerated by the cardiac tissue. Therefore, the administered dose of radiotherapy is usually infra-therapeutic for the cardiac angiosarcoma, trying to avoid excess of toxicity in the healthy cardiac tissue. Trying to increase the efficacy of this low dose of radiotherapy, combination with chemotherapy (chemo-radiotherapy) has been employed, looking for a better local control of the disease. The chemotherapy regimen employed for its combination with radiotherapy is usually carboplatin/paclitaxel or docetaxel. The combination of cardiac radiotherapy with cardiotoxic drugs as anthracyclines is not recommended [4].

- Look Hong et al. presented a case series of 18 patients [8]. Of the eight patients with localized/locally advanced disease, two received chemotherapy followed by surgery and intraoperative radiotherapy, one received chemotherapy alone, and one died before radiotherapy. Median overall survival was 13 months for the entire cohort; with median overall survival of 19.5 months for those presenting with localized/ locally advanced disease.
- Other case reported by Hata et al. showed the benefit of neoadjuvant chemo-radiotherapy with carboplatin and paclitaxel [17]. The authors presented a 40 years old man with lung metastases, and therefore unresectable, from a primary cardiac angiosarcoma. After six weeks of radiotherapy (radiation field limited to the primary cardiac tumour) combined with weekly paclitaxel and carboplatin a very good response both in the lung lesions and the primary malignancy was obtained with no progressive disease in the following 5 months.

When using systemic chemotherapy alone, some clarifications need to be made.

On the first hand, no much data are available for the management of primary cardiac angiosarcoma due to its poor survival and low incidence. Therefore, data from other soft tissue sarcoma are employed for the management of metastatic cardiac angiosarcomas [18].

On the second hand, angiosarcoma is a different entity of soft tissue sarcomas due to its high content in vascular involvement and angiogenesis. Several biological capabilities acquired during the multistep development of human tumours have been described during the last decades: sustaining proliferative signaling, evading growth suppressors, resisting cell death, enabling replicative immortality, inducing angiogenesis and activating invasion and metastasis [19]. Similar to Kaposi sarcomas, cardiac angiosarcomas arise from the endothelial cells, being one of the most important acquired capabilities the creation of new blood vessels [20]. Therefore, angiogenesis inhibitors have been of interest in the development of therapies for these tumours [21].

1. Chemotherapy Schedules According to the Data for Soft Tissue Sarcomas

Doxorubicin single agent or doxorubicin based combinations are the first line treatment for soft tissues sarcomas.

Others active drugs like gemcitabine, ifosfamide or docetaxel can also be employed. The sensitivity of soft tissue sarcomas to systemic doxorrubicin was demonstrated 40 years ago. A relationship between the dose and the effectiveness seems to exist: the optimal activity appears with ≥60 mg/m^2 per cycle, usually administered once every three weeks [22].

2. Chemotherapy Schedules with "Antiangiogenic Effect": Weekly Taxanes, Pegylated-Liposomal Doxorubicin

In addition to cancer cells, conventional cytotoxic chemotherapeutics also affect the endothelium of the growing tumour vasculature. This anti-angiogenic effect seems to be related to the administration of low doses of drug on a frequent or continuous schedule, known as 'metronomic' chemotherapy [23]. Weekly taxanes is an example of this "metronomic" chemotherapy with anti-angiogenic effect.

The liposomal encapsulation of pegylated liposomal-doxorubicin (PLD) seems to improve the side effect profile of doxorubicin. Studies in soft tissues sarcomas have proved the similar efficacy of doxorubicin (75 mg/m^2 every 3 weeks) compared with PLD (50 mg/m^2 every 4 weeks) [24]. However, PLD seem to have an extra anti-angiogenic effect. PLD is a large liposome with polyethylene glycol anchored within the lipid bilayer, which acts as a hydrophilic coating to prolong the circulating half-life of the liposome. Therefore, the degradation within the reticuloendothelial system is avoided producing a metronomic absorption of the chemotherapy: this is the postulated mechanism for the anti-angiogenesis effect of the PLD.

Paclitaxel, has been widely employed for the management of angiosarcomas [25-28]. A multicenter retrospective analysis of 32 patients showed its effectiveness in angiosarcomas: paclitaxel could be administered both every three weeks or in a weekly schedule [25]. The median time to progression was 7.6 months (range, 1-42) for the whole group. This results were confirmed in the Angiotax study, a prospective phase II trial with intravenous weekly paclitaxel (dose of 80 mg/m^2 on days 1, 8, and 15 of a 4-week cycle) [26]. Thirty patients with locally advanced/metastatic angiosarcoma were entered into the Angiotax study. The progression-free survival rates after 2 and 4 months were 74% and 45%, respectively. The median time to progression was 4 months and the median overall survival was 8 months.

Italiano et al. published a retrospective analysis of 117 metastastic angiosarcomas [20]. The aim of the analysis was to compare the results with doxorubicin and weekly paclitaxel. Seventy-five patients were treated with weekly paclitaxel and 42 with single-agent doxorubicin. Median overall survival of all the series was 8.5 months (95% CI, 6.4-10.7 months). In this study, first-line single-agent doxorubicin and weekly paclitaxel seem to have similar efficacy in metastatic angiosarcomas.

A small series of nine patients with cutaneous angiosarcoma were treated with systemic weekly docetaxel (25 mg/m^2) [29]. Six of the 9 patients achieved major responses, including

2 complete responses and 4 partial responses. The authors concluded that docetaxel could be effective in patients with cutaneous angisarcoma.

Good results in case reports and small series have been reported with PLD [30, 31]. Eight patients diagnosed with cutaneous angiosarcoma were treated with PLD [30]. The treatment was well tolerated with high rate of responses and a potencial way of increasing the sensitivity to subsequent radiation therapy.

A retrospective analysis of 14 patients diagnosed with metastatic angiosarcoma was published by Skubitz et al. The aim of the analysis was to compare the efficacy of the treatment with weekly paclitaxel and the treatment with pegylated-liposomal doxorubicin [32]. This study showed activity with both, pegylated-liposomal doxorubicin (five of six patients experienced clinical benefit) and paclitaxel in angiosarcoma.

Therefore, putting all the data together, first line chemotherapy with rather PLD or weekly paclitaxel are consider the standard of care for patients with metastatic angiosarcoma.

3. Target Therapies: Inhibiting Angiogenesis

However, apart from the standard chemotherapy (see above), target therapies focused on the intracellular pathways related with the creation and maintenance of these malignancies are also been explored. The main druggable target involved in angiosarcoma, seems to be the angiogenesis.

Angiogenesis is a complex process under both positive and negative control by naturally-occurring growth factors. Table 1 summarizes the most important treatments and targets for anti-angiogenic treatment. Few of them have been developed in angiosarcomas even it seems to be an important pathway to inhibit [33].

Bevacizumab is a monoclonal antibody targeting VEGF. VEGF-pathway was shown to be relevant in angiosarcomas in preclinical studies [34-36]. With those data, a phase II trial was completed with 32 patients receiving bevacizumab 15 mg/kg in 21-days cycles [37]. 17% of the patients had a partial response and 50% showed stable disease with a mean time to progression of 26 weeks. With these results, several studies are now ongoing, studying the efficacy of bevacizumab in angiosarcomas:

- Two new phase II trials are recruiting patients combining bevacizumab with weekly paclitaxel (AngioTaxPlus study (NCT01303497(38)) and NCT0155028(38))
- Other phase II will study the combination of gemcitabine, docetaxel and bevaciumab in selected soft tissue sarcomas, including angiosarcomas (NCT00887809(38)).

Sorafenib is a tyrosine kinase inhibitor with anti-angiogenic effect. Forty-one patients diagnosed with angiosarcoma received sorafenib (400 mg twice daily) for 9 months until unacceptable toxicity or tumour progression in context of a phase II study [39]. The results were better in the cutaneous angiosarcoma subgroup. In those patients diagnosed with a non-cutaneous angiosarcoma the progression-free rate at 9 months of treatment was 0% with median overall survival of 9 months.

Sunitinib, as sorafenib, is a tyrosine kinase inhibitor. A phase II trial with non-GIST soft tissue sarcomas was completed [40]. Two angiosarcomas were included in this study and the dose of sunitinib was 37.5 mg daily. Patients´ response was reassessed with FDG-PET: metabolic stable disease was seen in 11 (52%) of 21 patients.

Other two tyrosine kinase inhibitors are now recruiting patients in two phase II trial with angiosarcoma: axitinib (NCT01140737(38)) and pazopanib (NCT01462630(38)). Other phase II will study the treatment with gemcitabine with or without pazopanib for second line treatment of soft tissue sarcomas (NCT01532687(38)).

Table 1.

Drug	Target
Tyrosine kinase inhibitors with anti-angiogenic effect	
Sunitinib	c-kit, VEGFR1-3, PDGFRa, PDGFRb, FLT3, CSF-1R, and REarranged during Transfection (RET)
Sorafenib	VEGFR2, fms-like tyrosine kinase 3 (FLT3), PDGFR, and fibroblast growth factor receptor (FGFR)-1
Pazopanib	VEGFR1-3, PDGFR alpha and beta, FGFR1 and 3, c-kit,
Cediranib	VEGFR
Vandetanib	VEGFR, RET, and EGFR
Axitinib	VEGFR inhibitor that targets VEGFR1-3
Regorafenib	VEGFR1-3 in addition to RET, c-kit, PDGFRa and b, FGFR1 and 2, and other membrane-bound and intracellular kinases
Monoclonal antibodies anti-angiogenic pathway	
Bevacizumab	VEGF-A
Aflibercept	VEGF-A, VEGF-B, and PIGF
Others antiangiogenic approaches	
Thalidomide, lenalidomida	Inmunomodulatory drugs
Interferon	
Cixutumumab	IGF-R inhibitor
Erlotinib, Gefitinib, Cetuximab	EGF-EGFR pathway inhibitors
EZN-2968	Hipoxia-inducible factors inhibition
RO4929097	Notch pathway inhibitor
Demcizumab (anti DLL4)	
Everolimus, Temsirolimus	Rapamycin analog, inhibition of mTOR
REGN910 and Trebananib	Angiopoietins inhibitors (anti-Tie2 tyrosine kinase inhibitors)
Aspirin, Celecoxib	COX-2 inhibitors

Cixutumumab is a monoclonal antibody inhibiting IGF-R. The expression of IGF-R has been previously studied in sarcomas and is known its relation with the angiogenesis [41]. Therefore, one phase I trial is ongoing, recruiting patients with soft tissue sarcoma, studying the safety of the combination of cixutumumab and doxorubicin (NCT00720174(38)).

Other phase I/II trial is ongoing recruiting patients with soft tissue sarcomas for treatment with Vismodegib (Hedgehog inhibitor) combined with gamma-secretase/Notch signalling pathway inhibitor RO4929097 (Notch inhibitor) (NCT01154452(38)).

The expression of angiopoietin-TIE system has been the aim of several preclinical studies [42]. The authors evaluated immunohistochemically human angiosarcoma samples looking for the impact in prognosis of the expression of angiopoietin-1, angiopoietin-2, TIE1 and TEK (TIE2) proteins. Moderate to strong expression of angiopoietin-1, TIE1 and TEK (TIE2) was identified in the majority of angiosarcomas and moderate to strong expression of angiopoietin-2 was observed in 42% of them. The expression of angiopoietin-1 correlated with survival and the expression of angiopoietin-2, TIE1 and TEK (TIE2) was associated with vasoformative architecture. Authors concluded that reduced expression of these proteins was associated with non-vasoformative and clinically more aggressive lesions.

With the development of drugs able to inhibit TIE2, Hasenstein et al. reported their results with xenograft modelling using cell lines of angiosarcoma [43]. TIE2 inhibition seemed to delay tumour growth by increasing tumour cell apoptosis. Clinical studies are awaited, with an ongoing phase II trial with trebananib recruiting patients with angiosarcoma (NCT01623869(38)).

After having benefit in a case report [44], a prospective study was completed with razoxane, visdesine and radiation. According to the known effect of razoxane leading to a redifferentiation of pathological tumour blood vessels, there was interest of studing its effect in angiosarcoma. A phase II trial with 13 patients was performed [45]. From nine patients with measurable vascular soft tissue sarcomas (eight angiosarcomas and one hemangiopericytoma), 6 complete remissions, 2 partial remissions and 1 minor remission were achieved: a major response rate of 89%. More studies are awaited.

Interferon (IFN) is an immunomodulation treatment widely employed in other malignancies as melanoma and neuroendocrine tumours. Treatment with interferon has shown activity in some case reports: patients were treated with intralesional IFN for cutaneous angiosarcomas, combined with doxorubicin or radiotherapy [46-48]. A preclinical study analyzed the effect of IFN in mice models of angiosarcoma [49]. The authors concluded that the antitumour effects of IFN-alpha were likely mediated through angiogenesis inhibition rather than solely by direct inhibition of tumour cell proliferation.

Finally, the inhibition of mTOR pathway, also with angiogenic effect, can be inhibited with the everolimus or temsirolimus. Encouraging preclinical data were published in 2013 [50]. The authors investigated mechanistic (mammalian) target of rapamycin (mTOR) signaling in benign and malignant vascular tumours, and the effects of mTOR kinase inhibitor as a potential therapy for these lesions using human vascular tumours (infantile hemangioma and angiosarcoma). Phosphorylation of p70 S6-kinase (S6K) and S6 ribosomal protein (S6), which are activated downstream of mTOR complex-1 (mTORC1), were analyzed by immunohistochemical stains and western blot. Vascular tumours showed increased activation of S6K and S6. Rapamycin significantly reduced vascular tumour growth in vitro and in vivo. Similar results were shown in other preclinical study, revealing the importance of mTOR signaling pathways in benign and malignant vascular tumours and the potential benefit of employing mTOR inhibition in these patients [51]. According to the literature available, two patients diagnosed with angiosarcoma have been treated with combination of paclitaxel and everolimus in context of a phase I clinical trial [52]. No data of efficacy are available yet for this combination. More studies are awaited.

To summarize, the available data for the treatment with angiosarcoma are few, with no specific studies for cardiac angiosarcoma due to its rarity and poor prognosis. However, the results with anti-angiogenic chemotherapy as PLD or weekly paclitaxel are encouraging. Therefore, rather PLD or weekly paclitaxel, are considered the first line treatment for metastatic angiosarcoma. Lot of effort is being done during the last decade with preclinical studies and small prospective studies looking for new target therapies for this patients focusing in the inhibition of the angiogenesis. The future looks promising even lot of work needs still to be done.

Conflict of interest

Angela Lamarca is funded by ESMO Fellowship program. No conflict of interest.

References

[1] Fury, M. G., Antonescu, C. R., Van Zee, K. J., Brennan, M. F., Maki, R. G. A 14-year retrospective review of angiosarcoma: clinical characteristics, prognostic factors, and treatment outcomes with surgery and chemotherapy. *Cancer J.* 2005; 11(3):241-247.

[2] Mark, R. J., Poen, J. C., Tran, L. M., Fu, Y. S., Juillard, G. F. Angiosarcoma. A report of 67 patients and a review of the literature. *Cancer* 1996; 77(11):2400-2406.

[3] Patel, R. M., Billings, S. D. Cutaneous soft tissue tumors that make you say, "oh $*and%!". *Adv. Anat. Pathol.* 2012; 19(5):320-330.

[4] Bouma, W., Lexis, C. P., Willems, T. P., Suurmeijer, A. J., van dH, I, Ebels, T., et al. Successful surgical excision of primary right atrial angiosarcoma. *J. Cardiothorac. Surg.* 2011; 6:47.

[5] Bruce, C. J. Cardiac tumours: diagnosis and management. *Heart* 2011; 97(2):151-160.

[6] Burke, A., Jeudy, J., Jr., Virmani, R. Cardiac tumours: an update: Cardiac tumours. *Heart* 2008; 94(1):117-123.

[7] Kodali, D., Seetharaman, K. Primary cardiac angiosarcoma. *Sarcoma* 2006; 2006: 39130.

[8] Look Hong, N. J., Pandalai, P. K., Hornick, J. L., Shekar, P. S., Harmon, D. C., Chen, Y. L., et al. Cardiac Angiosarcoma Management and Outcomes: 20-Year Single-institution Experience. *Ann. Surg. Oncol.* 2012; 19(8):2707-2715.

[9] Grebenc, M. L., Rosado de Christenson, M. L., Burke, A. P., Green, C. E., Galvin, J. R. Primary cardiac and pericardial neoplasms: radiologic-pathologic correlation. *Radiographics* 2000; 20(4):1073-1103.

[10] Burke, A. P., Cowan, D., Virmani, R. Primary sarcomas of the heart. *Cancer* 1992; 69 (2):387-395.

[11] Randall, M. B., Geisinger, K. R. Angiosarcoma of the heart: pericardial fluid cytology. *Diagn. Cytopathol.* 1990; 6(1):58-62.

[12] Ge, Y., Ro, J. Y., Kim, D., Kim, C. H., Reardon, M. J., Blackmon, S., et al. Clinicopathologic and immunohistochemical characteristics of adult primary cardiac angiosarcomas: analysis of 10 cases. *Ann. Diagn. Pathol.* 2011; 15(4):262-267.

[13] Grandmougin, D., Fayad, G., Decoene, C., Pol, A., Warembourg, H. Total orthotopic heart transplantation for primary cardiac rhabdomyosarcoma: factors influencing long-term survival. *Ann. Thorac. Surg.* 2001; 71(5):1438-1441.

[14] Slepicka, C., Durci, M. Cardiac angiosarcoma treated with resection and adjuvant radiation therapy. *J. La State Med. Soc.* 2012; 164(2):92-93.

[15] Llombart-Cussac, A., Pivot, X., Contesso, G., Rhor-Alvarado, A., Delord, J. P., Spielmann, M., et al. Adjuvant chemotherapy for primary cardiac sarcomas: the IGR experience. *Br. J. Cancer* 1998; 78(12):1624-1628.

[16] Pigott, C., Welker, M., Khosla, P., Higgins, R. S. Improved outcome with multimodality therapy in primary cardiac angiosarcoma. *Nat. Clin. Pract. Oncol.* 2008; 5(2):112-115.

[17] Hata, A., Katakami, N., Fujita, S., Kokubo, M., Imai, Y. Angiosarcoma arising from right atrium: remarkable response to concurrent chemoradiotherapy with carboplatin and paclitaxel. *J. Thorac. Oncol.* 2011; 6(5):970-971.

[18] Penel, N., Marreaud, S., Robin, Y. M., Hohenberger, P. Angiosarcoma: state of the art and perspectives. *Crit. Rev. Oncol. Hematol.* 2011; 80(2):257-263.

[19] Hanahan, D., Weinberg, R. A. Hallmarks of cancer: the next generation. *Cell* 2011; 144 (5):646-674.

[20] Italiano, A., Cioffi, A., Penel, N., Levra, M. G., Delcambre, C., Kalbacher, E., et al. Comparison of doxorubicin and weekly paclitaxel efficacy in metastatic angiosarcomas. *Cancer* 2012; 118(13):3330-3336.

[21] Young, R. J., Brown, N. J., Reed, M. W., Hughes, D., Woll, P. J. Angiosarcoma. *Lancet Oncol.* 2010; 11(10):983-991.

[22] Borden, E. C., Amato, D. A., Rosenbaum, C., Enterline, H. T., Shiraki, M. J., Creech, R. H., et al. Randomized comparison of three adriamycin regimens for metastatic soft tissue sarcomas. *J. Clin. Oncol.* 1987; 5(6):840-850.

[23] Kerbel, R. S., Kamen, B. A. The anti-angiogenic basis of metronomic chemotherapy. *Nat. Rev. Cancer* 2004; 4(6):423-436.

[24] Judson, I., Radford, J. A., Harris, M., Blay, J. Y., van Hoesel, Q., Le Cesne, A., et al. Randomised phase II trial of pegylated liposomal doxorubicin (DOXIL/CAELYX) versus doxorubicin in the treatment of advanced or metastatic soft tissue sarcoma: a study by the EORTC Soft Tissue and Bone Sarcoma Group. *Eur. J. Cancer* 2001; 37 (7):870-877.

[25] Schlemmer, M., Reichardt, P., Verweij, J., Hartmann, J. T., Judson, I., Thyss, A., et al. Paclitaxel in patients with advanced angiosarcomas of soft tissue: a retrospective study of the EORTC soft tissue and bone sarcoma group. *Eur. J. Cancer* 2008; 44(16):2433-2436.

[26] Penel, N., Bui, B. N., Bay, J. O., Cupissol, D., Ray-Coquard, I., Piperno-Neumann, S., et al. Phase II trial of weekly paclitaxel for unresectable angiosarcoma: the ANGIOTAX Study. *J. Clin. Oncol.* 2008; 26(32):5269-5274.

[27] Fata, F., O'Reilly, E., Ilson, D., Pfister, D., Leffel, D., Kelsen, D. P., et al. Paclitaxel in the treatment of patients with angiosarcoma of the scalp or face. *Cancer* 1999; 86(10): 2034-2037.

[28] Ram Prabu, M. P., Thulkar, S., Ray, R., Bakhshi, S. Primary cardiac angiosarcoma with good response to Paclitaxel. *J. Thorac. Oncol.* 2011; 6(10):1778-1779.

[29] Nagano, T., Yamada, Y., Ikeda, T., Kanki, H., Kamo, T., Nishigori, C. Docetaxel: a therapeutic option in the treatment of cutaneous angiosarcoma: report of 9 patients. *Cancer* 2007; 110(3):648-651.

[30] Wollina, U., Hansel, G., Schonlebe, J., Averbeck, M., Paasch, U., Uhl, J., et al. Cutaneous angiosarcoma is a rare aggressive malignant vascular tumour of the skin. *J. Eur. Acad. Dermatol. Venereol.* 2011; 25(8):964-968.

[31] Eiling, S., Lischner, S., Busch, J. O., Rothaupt, D., Christophers, E., Hauschild, A. Complete remission of a radio-resistant cutaneous angiosarcoma of the scalp by systemic treatment with liposomal doxorubicin. *Br. J. Dermatol.* 2002; 147(1):150-153.

[32] Skubitz, K. M., Haddad, P. A. Paclitaxel and pegylated-liposomal doxorubicin are both active in angiosarcoma. *Cancer* 2005; 104(2):361-366.

[33] Park, M. S., Ravi, V., Araujo, D. M. Inhibiting the VEGF-VEGFR pathway in angiosarcoma, epithelioid hemangioendothelioma, and hemangiopericytoma/solitary fibrous tumor. *Curr. Opin. Oncol.* 2010; 22(4):351-355.

[34] Stacher, E., Gruber-Mosenbacher, U., Halbwedl, I., Dei Tos, A. P., Cavazza, A., Papotti, M. et al. The VEGF-system in primary pulmonary angiosarcomas and haemangioendotheliomas: new potential therapeutic targets? *Lung Cancer* 2009; 65(1): 49-55.

[35] Arbiser, J. L., Larsson, H., Claesson-Welsh, L., Bai, X., LaMontagne, K., Weiss, S. W., et al. Overexpression of VEGF 121 in immortalized endothelial cells causes conversion to slowly growing angiosarcoma and high level expression of the VEGF receptors VEGFR-1 and VEGFR-2 in vivo. *Am. J. Pathol.* 2000; 156(4):1469-1476.

[36] Tokuyama, W., Mikami, T., Masuzawa, M., Okayasu, I. Autocrine and paracrine roles of VEGF/VEGFR-2 and VEGF-C/VEGFR-3 signaling in angiosarcomas of the scalp and face. *Hum. Pathol.* 2010; 41(3):407-414.

[37] Agulnik, M., Yarber, J. L., Okuno, S. H., von Mehren, M., Jovanovic, B. D., Brockstein, B. E., et al. An open-label, multicenter, phase II study of bevacizumab for the treatment of angiosarcoma and epithelioid hemangioendotheliomas. *Ann. Oncol.* 2012.

[38] http://www.clinicaltrials.gov/. 2013.

[39] Ray-Coquard, I., Italiano, A., Bompas, E., Le Cesne, A., Robin, Y. M., Chevreau, C., et al. Sorafenib for patients with advanced angiosarcoma: a phase II Trial from the French Sarcoma Group (GSF/GETO). *Oncologist* 2012; 17(2):260-266.

[40] George, S., Merriam, P., Maki, R. G., Van den Abbeele, A. D., Yap, J. T., Akhurst, T., et al. Multicenter phase II trial of sunitinib in the treatment of nongastrointestinal stromal tumor sarcomas. *J. Clin. Oncol.* 2009; 27(19):3154-3160.

[41] Roholl, P. J., Skottner, A., Prinsen, I., Lips, C. J., Den Otter, W., Van Unnik, J. A. Expression of insulin-like growth factor 1 in sarcomas. *Histopathology* 1990; 16(5): 455-460.

[42] Buehler, D., Rush, P., Hasenstein, J. R., Rice, S. R., Hafez, G. R., Longley, B. J., et al. Expression of angiopoietin-TIE system components in angiosarcoma. *Mod. Pathol.* 2013; 26(8):1032-1040.

[43] Hasenstein, J. R., Kasmerchak, K., Buehler, D., Hafez, G. R., Cleary, K., Moody, J. S., et al. Efficacy of Tie2 receptor antagonism in angiosarcoma. *Neoplasia* 2012; 14(2): 131-140.

[44] Rhomberg, W., Grass, M. [Angiosarcoma of the right atrium: local control via low radiation doses and razoxane. A case report]. *Strahlenther Onkol.* 1999; 175(3):102-104.

[45] Rhomberg, W., Wink, A., Pokrajac, B., Eiter, H., Hackl, A., Pakisch, B., et al. Treatment of vascular soft tissue sarcomas with razoxane, vindesine, and radiation. *Int. J. Radiat. Oncol. Biol. Phys.* 2009; 74(1):187-191.

[46] Jackel, A., Deichmann, M., Waldmann, V., Bock, M., Naher, H. Regression of metastatic angiosarcoma of the skin after systemic treatment with liposome-encapsulated doxorubicin and interferon-alpha. *Br. J. Dermatol.* 1999; 140(6):1187-1188.

[47] Ulrich, L., Krause, M., Brachmann, A., Franke, I., Gollnick, H. Successful treatment of angiosarcoma of the scalp by intralesional cytokine therapy and surface irradiation. *J. Eur. Acad. Dermatol. Venereol.* 2000; 14(5):412-415.

[48] Bong, A. B., Bonnekoh, B., Schon, M. P., Gollnick, H. Treatment of scalp angiosarcoma by controlled perfusion of A. carotis externa with pegylated liposomal doxorubicin and intralesional application of pegylated interferon alfa. *J. Am. Acad. Dermatol.* 2005; 52(2 Suppl. 1):20-23.

[49] Taylor, K. L., Oates, R. K., Grane, R., Leaman, D. W., Borden, E. C., Lindner, D. J. IFN-alpha1,8 inhibits tumor-induced angiogenesis in murine angiosarcomas. *J. Interferon. Cytokine Res.* 2006; 26(5):353-361.

[50] Du, W., Gerald, D., Perruzzi, C. A., Rodriguez-Waitkus, P., Enayati, L., Krishnan, B., et al. Vascular tumors have increased p70 S6-kinase activation and are inhibited by topical rapamycin. *Lab. Invest.* 2013.

[51] M Wada MHTSMMNK. Targeting PI3K/mTOR signaling in cutaneous angiosarcoma. *Journal of Investigative Dermatology* (2013)133,S56-S76.doi:10.1038/jid.2013.96. 2013.

[52] Campone, M., Levy, V., Bourbouloux, E., Berton, R. D., Bootle, D., Dutreix, C., et al. Safety and pharmacokinetics of paclitaxel and the oral mTOR inhibitor everolimus in advanced solid tumours. *Br. J. Cancer* 2009; 100(2):315-321.

In: Rare Diseases
Editors: Giorgio Di Giovanni and Pietro Marcoz
ISBN: 978-1-62948-525-6

Chapter VII

Clear Cell Adenocarcinoma of the Bladder: Diagnosis and Management

***Ji Lu*[1], *Zhihui Xu*[2] *and Chunxi Wang*[1*]**
[1]Department of Urology, The First Hospital of Jilin University, Changchun, China
[2]The Key Laboratory of Pathobiology, Ministry of Education, College of Basic Medical Sciences, Jilin University, Changchun, China

Abstract

Clear cell adenocarcinoma (CCA) is an extremely rare variant of adenocarcinoma of the bladder. In contrast to the common urothelial carcinoma of the bladder, CCA affects women more often than men. Since it was first reported in 1968, only a few reports have been available on this rare disease. Accurate recognition and diagnosis for clear cell adenocarcinoma of the bladder is difficult due to its rarity and uncharacteristic clinical presentation. Moreover, it is relatively more malignant with poor prognosis than the common urothelial carcinoma. Experiences are still accumulating in treating this disease. In this review, we characterized clinical aspects of clear cell adenocarcinoma of the bladder, including epidemiology, clinical presentation, diagnosis, treatment and prognosis. This may help the clinicians to recognize and diagnose this rare bladder carcinoma, and formulate treatment recommendations.

Keywords: Clear cell adenocarcinoma, bladder, diagnosis, treatment

Introduction

Clear cell adenocarcinoma of the bladder is an extremely rare variant of bladder adenocarcinoma. Based on the definition of World Health Organization, bladder adenocarcinoma is a malignant neoplasm derived from the urothelium showing histologically

* Corresponding Author address Email: chunxi_wang@126.com.

pure glandular phenotype [1]. Clear cell type is one of its histological growth patterns. Other patterns include enteric (colonic) type, adenocarcinoma not otherwise specified (NOS), signet ring cell, mucinous (colloid), hepatoid and mixed [1]. The disease was first reported by Dow and Young in 1968 [2]. CCA of the bladder is relatively more malignant with poor prognosis than the urothelial carcinoma of bladder. Current knowledge of this disease is limited due to few studies have been conducted on this rare disease. In this review, we searched relevant case reports published in English literatures. To better evaluate clinical characteristics of this disease, the case reports that do not have any data about demography or treatment outcomes are excluded. In this review, we summarized clinical aspects of clear cell adenocarcinoma of the bladder, including epidemiology, clinical presentation, diagnosis, treatment and prognosis.

Epidemiology

Bladder cancer is the most common malignancy of the urinary tract, and the 9th most common cancer diagnosis worldwide, with more than 330,000 new cases each year and more than 130,000 deaths per year. It is generally estimated male:female incidence ratio is 3.8:1.0 [3]. The histological and pathological type of bladder cancer is mainly urothelial carcinoma, also called transitional cell carcinoma (TCC), accounting for approximately 90% of total bladder carcinoma cases [4].

Other types of bladder carcinoma, including squamous cell carcinoma and adenocarcinoma, account for 3-7% and <2%, respectively[5]. As an extremely rare variant of bladder adenocarcinoma, some demographic characteristics of the clear cell type are distinct from those in patients with TCC. The majority of patients are female. Base on current case reports the mean sex ratio is about 2:1 (Female=39, Male =20, NA =1). Most patients are in the fifth to seventh decade at the time of first diagnosis. The mean age is 60.7, ranging from 35 to 83. Table 1 summarizes the epidemiological and clinical characteristics of CCA of the bladder.

Clinical Features

The clinical features of CCA of the bladder are similar to those of common TCC and reflect the presence of a tumoral mass. Gross hematuria is the most common symptom in CCA, which accounted for about 58.3% (14/24). Dysuria has been reported as the second most common symptom (45.8%, 11/24).

Other symptoms, such as urinary tract infection, increased urinary frequency, urgency, and urinary retention, have been occasionally reported. Patients rarely complained of local tumor effects or pain from local spread of the tumor. Based on available data, the most common locations which tumors originated from were bladder neck, trigone and posterior wall. Other common locations included anterior, lateral, and superior bladder wall, diverticulum, and urethra. Unlike urothelial carcinoma, most clear cell adenocarcinomas of bladder were large, solitary masses forming papillary or sessile structures with the size ranging from 0.4cm to 7.4cm.

Table 1. Demographics and clinical characteristics of patients with CCA of the bladder

References	Age	Sex	Symptoms	Sites	Size (cm)
Dow 1968 [2]	43	M	Urinary frequency, urgency and tenesmus, gross hematuria	Right lateral wall, neck, prostatic urethra	NA
Skor,1977 [6]	54	F	Dysuria, suprapubic pain, urgency, urinary retention	Neck	NA
Schultz, 1984 [7]	70	F	Urinary urgency and frequency	Trigone	3.0x6.0
Young, 1985 [8]	78	F	Gross hematuria, frequency, dysuria	Trigone	2.5x2.0x0.4
Chore, 1993 [9]	35	F	hematuria	Posterior wall	NA
Doria, 1996 [10]	45	F	painless hematuria	Trigone	8.0x5.0x2.2
Doria, 1996 [10]	63	M	hematuria	right wall of bladder	2.5x2.0x1.8
Drew, 1996 [11]	63	M	NA	NA	NA
Drew, 1996 [11]	78	F	NA	NA	NA
Drew, 1996 [11]	50	M	NA	NA	NA
Drew, 1996 [11]	43	M	NA	NA	NA
Mai, 2000 [12]	68	F	NA	Diverticulum, right side of upper part of trigone	3.0x3.0x2.7
Matsuoka, 2002 [13]	64	F	NA	Neck	NA
Matsuoka, 2002 [13]	71	F	NA	Neck, urethra	NA
Matsuoka, 2002 [13]	53	F	NA	Right ureteral orifice	NA
Matsuoka, 2002 [13]	68	F	NA	Posterior, left lateral wall	NA
Matsuoka, 2002 [13]	NA	NA	NA	NA	NA
Matsuoka, 2002 [13]	63	M	NA	Left lateral wall, trigone	NA
Matsuoka, 2002 [13]	57	F	NA	Neck	NA
Matsuoka, 2002 [13]	61	F	NA	Posterior wall	NA
Matsuoka, 2002 [13]	62	F	NA	Left ureteral orifice	NA

Table 1. (Continued)

References	Age	Sex	Symptoms	Sites	Size (cm)
Matsuoka,2002 [13]	62	F	NA	Posterior wall, trigone	NA
Matsuoka, 2002 [13]	73	F	NA	Posterior, anterior wall, neck, urethra	NA
Matsuoka, 2002 [13]	53	M	NA	Posterior, anterior wall	NA
Matsuoka, 2002 [13]	78	F	NA	Right lateral wall, neck	NA
Matsuoka, 2002 [13]	72	M	NA	Trigone, posterior, left lateral wall	NA
Matsuoka, 2002 [13]	67	M	NA	trigone, posterior wall	NA
Matsuoka, 2002 [13]	80	M	NA	neck, left ureteral orifice	NA
Matsuoka, 2002 [13]	65	M	NA	anterior wall	NA
Matsuoka, 2002 [13]	59	F	NA	trigone, neck	NA
Matsuoka, 2002 [13]	59	M	Oliguria, left lower abdominal pain, loss of appetite, increased urinary frequency	posterior wall	5.0x5.0x3.0
Oliva, 2002 [14]	22-83	11F,2M	Hematuria, terminal dysuria and urinary obstruction in two, urinary urgency and incontinence in one	trigone, posterior or left wall of the bladder	1.0-7.0cm
Moinzadeh, 2003 [15]	69	M	Gross intermittent hematuria	Diverticulum, right ureteral orifice	5.0
Signori, 2003	54	M	Painless gross haematuria	done of bladder	2.5x2.0
Kosem, 2005	55	M	Dysuria, painless hematuria with clots	Left lateral wall	NA
Kurosaka, 2005	52	F	NA	Trigone, bilateral iliac lymphadenopathy	4.0x3.0x3.0
Lum, 2006	68	M	Recurrent UTI, chronic urinary retention	NA	NA

References	Age	Sex	Symptoms	Sites	Size (cm)
Adams, 2007	62	F	UTI, dysuria, intermittent hematuria	neck, trigone, urethra, right lymph node	3.8
Sun, 2008	69	M	Dysuria, painless hematuria	NA	NA
Sun, 2008	56	F	Lower urinary tract symptoms, microscopic hematuria	NA	NA
Pena Alvarez, 2010	49	F	mictional symptoms	Bladder neck, Left half of the trigone	NA
Rotellini, 2010	82	M	No particular symptoms	NA	6.5x3.0x2.0
Sethi, 2011	74	F	Obstructive and irritative lower urinary tract symptoms	Bladder neck, anterior and posterior walls	4.0x3.0x2.0
Lu, 2012	68	F	microscopic hematuria, dysuria, anemia	posterior wall, neck, urethra	6.4x7.4
Szymanski, 2012	50	F	gross hematuria, dysuria, urgency, frequency, pelvic discomfort	left lateral posterior bladder wall	4.6x3.5
Abbas, 2013	46	F	gross hematuria	NA	>3.0
Lah, 2013	59	F	intermittent hematuria	superior bladder wall	3.6x2.4x2.8
Terada, 2013	73	F	Renal failure, cardiac failure; hydronephrosis, hydroureter	NA	5.0x4.0x3.0

Abbreviations: NA = not available.

Pathogenesis

The precise pathogenesis of clear cell adenocarcinoma of the bladder is still controversial. Some hypotheses were proposed to explain the origin of CCA in the bladder. (1). CCA of the bladder arises from mesonephric derivation. This theory is supported by the fact that many CCA tumors are located in the trigone and urethra [7, 11, 16]. Actually in the older literatures, CCA in most cases were designated "mesonephric adenocarcinoma". But it has been also reported that CCA tumors were located at the posterior and lateral walls of the bladder, which do not embryologically arise from mesonephric remnants. (2). CCA arises from mullerian elements in the bladder. It has been found that CCA were histogenetically identical to CCA arising in the female genital tract [17]. In some cases the neoplasms have been associated with vesical endometriosis or have arisen in mullerian duct cysts or remnants in the bladder [9, 18]. This has also been considered an explanation for the observation that female incidence is dominant in this disease. (3). CCA derives from urothelial carcinoma with glandular differentiation. Some studies presented evidence that concurrent urothelial carcinoma or urothelial carcinoma in situ was observed in the CCA cases, supporting an urothelial origin despite the morphologic resemblance to certain mullerian-derived tumors of the female genital tract [14, 19]. (4) CCA results from malignant transformation of nephrogenic adenoma. Some studies suggested that CCA may be associated with nephrogenic adenoma because they share some similar histological features, and the molecular evidence for transformation of nephrogenic metaplasia to clear cell adenocarcinoma is also available [20-22].

Diagnosis

Due to the non-specific clinical features, diagnosis of CCA is mainly accomplished via histopathological examination of specimens obtained by cystoscopy and transurethral resection of the bladder tumor (TUR-BT). Immunohistochemistry staining can help to establish the diagnosis. The use of urinary cytology and molecular genetics in diagnosing CCA is still limited.

Histopathology

Microscopically, most of the tumor cells are arranged in tubular glands, microcysts or fine papillae architecturally, partly in diffuse sheets or solid nests (Figure 1) [23]. The tubular glands and microcysts have different sizes and irregular shapes with eosinophilic and/or basophilic secretions. Most tumor cells are in cuboidal or columnar shape. Characteristic hobnail cells with abundant clear cytoplasm can be seen (Figure 2) [23]. Tumor cells show moderate to marked cytologic atypia with high mitotic rate. One study showed that mitotic figures averaged at 16 (range, 5-36; median, 15) per 10 HPF for CCA cases [24].

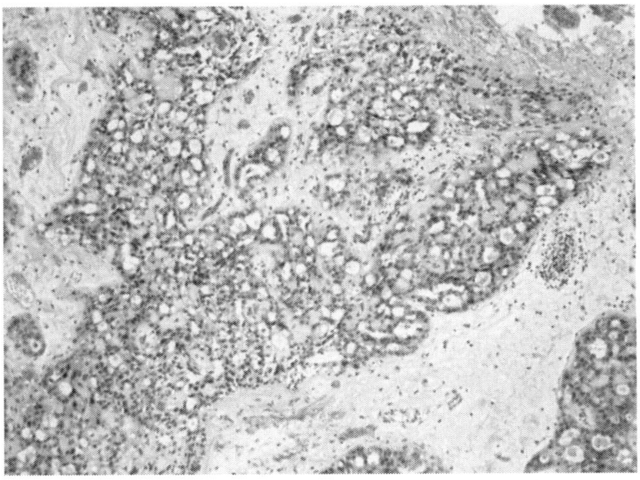

Figure 1. Clear cell adenocarcinoma of the bladder cells were arranged in tubular gland, microcysts or fine papillary in most area, partly in diffuse sheets or solid nests (Hematoxylin-eosin stain).

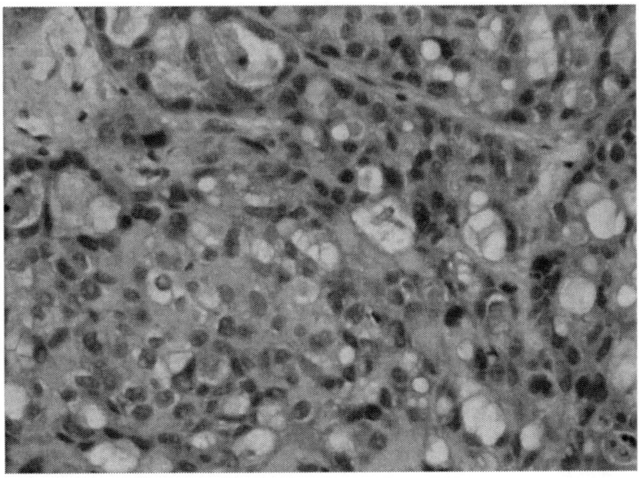

Figure 2. Clear cell adenocarcinoma of the bladder cells were in cuboidal, columnar or hobnail shape, with abundant clear cytoplasm. (Hematoxylin-eosin stain).

Immunohistochemistry

Immunohistochemistry has been the research focus for diagnosing clear cell adenocarcinoma of the lower urinary tract. Table 2 lists some markers that have been studied frequently in the immunohistochemistrical staining of CCA. CA125, CK7 and p53 have been shown to have high positive stain rates in most cases. They have 75-100%, 90-100% and 100% in a series of cases [11, 14, 19, 21, 25], and 87.5%(7/8), 88.9%(8/9) and 100%(3/3) in single cases [23, 26-34], respectively. ER, PR and PSA were demonstrated to be negative in all stuided cases [11, 14, 15, 21, 23, 26, 27, 32-34]. CK20 and CD10 have variable positive rate in CCA [14, 19, 23, 25-27, 29-32, 34]. Moreover, HNF-1β, GATA3 and PAX8 have been determined to be new markers for CCA in some series of cases through immunohistochemistry recently [30, 35, 36].

Table 2. Immunohistochemistry markers in clear cell adenocarcinoma of the bladder

Markers	CA-125	CK7	p53	CK20	CD10	ER	PR	PSA
series of cases								
Drew, 1996 [11] (n=6)	100% (6/6)							0% (0/6)
Glicrease, 1998 [21] (n=5)			100% (5/5)			0% (0/5)	0% (0/5)	0% (0/5)
Oliva, 2002 [14] (n=10)	100% (10/10)	90% (9/10)		50% (5/10)				0% (0/10)
Sun, 2008 [25] (n=4)	75% (3/4)	100% (4/4)		50% (2/4)				
Sung, 2008 [19] (n=12)		100% (10/12)		25% (3/12)	42% (5/12)			
single cases								
Signori, 2003 [34]		-		-				-
Moinzadeh, 2003 [15]								-
Kosem, 2005 [33]	+							-
Lum, 2006 [32]	+	+	+	+	-	-	-	-
Adams, 2007 [31]	-	+		-				
Rotellini, 2010 [30]		+		+	+			
Sethi, 2011 [29]	+	+	+	-				
Lu, 2012 [23]	+	+		+		-	-	
Szymanski, 2012 [28]	+	+						
Terada, 2013 [26]	+	+	+	-	+	-	-	
Abbas, 2013 [27]	+	+		+/-	+	-	-	-

Abbreviations: CA-125 = cancer antigen 125; CK7 = cytokeratine 7; CK20 = cytokeratine 20; ER = estrogen receptor; PR = progesterone receptor.

Urinary Cytology

The studies of urinary cytology in CCA of the bladder are limited. Cytomorphologic features included variably cellular samples with 3-dimensional fragments of malignant cells that had enlarged nuclei, prominent nucleoli, and occasional hobnail configurations. Some samples showed luminal formation with collection of neutrophils [37]. However, because the variable shedding of tumor cells into the urine, or other factors such as inflammation, hematuria, and cellular degeneration are involved in the urine, urine cytologic examination failed to detect tumor in some patients, or only atypical cells were found in some cases [15, 25]. Moreover, urothelial carcinoma, the most common malignancy of the bladder, is often the presumptive diagnosis. All this may lead to an incorrect diagnosis. Thus, the primary role of urinary cytology is to differentiate among benign, reactive, low-grade, and high-grade urothelial lesions, and it may not be able to distinguish rare malignant bladder neoplasms from urothelial carcinoma [28].

Molecular Genetics

Recent advances in molecular genetics have identified a variety of alterations of chromosomes, such as chromosomes 3, 7, 9, and 17, in urothelial carcinoma [38, 39]. However, few studies have been done in CCA of the lower urinary tract. Sung and collegues studied genetic alteration of CCA through UroVysion FISH assay, showing that gains of chromosomes 3 and 17 in all 12 tumors (100%), gains of chromosome 7 in 11 of 12 tumors (92%), and loss of chromosome 9p21 in 3 of 12 tumors (25%) [19]. In another study, Rotellini displayed the similar results through the same technique, showing polysomy of chromosomes 3, 7, and 17 without observation of 9p21 allele loss [30].

Differential Diagnosis

Although histopathology can help us to diagnose the clear cell adenocarcinoma of the bladder by characteristic histopathologic findings, such as clear cytoplasm, CCA of the bladder must be differentiated from several other cancers: CCA of gynecologic organs with bladder invasion, metastatic clear cell renal carcinoma, primary urothelial carcinoma with clear cell differentiation, and carcinoma arising from nephrogenic adenoma.

The first two diseases are relatively easy to exclude after thorough examination and history review. In a patient with an earlier clear cell renal cell carcinoma, GATA3 and UroVysion FISH assay have been used as a bladder cancer marker to elucidate the nonmetastatic origin of the bladder tumor with a clear cell feature [30].The latter two diseases are more difficult to distinguish. The primary urothelial carcinoma with clear cell differentiation may have abundant glycogen-rich clear cytoplasm, but its architecture is less variable. It lacks hobnail cells, and the clear cells appear more squamoid [21]. Differentiating CCA from nephrogenic adenoma can be based on some clinical and histologic features. Compared to nephrogenic adenoma (NA), which is regarded as a metaplastic lesion, CCA is a neoplasm. NA can be seen more often in men, wherease CCA occurs predominantly in older women. Most nephrogenic adenomas are associated with a history of genitorunary trauma, surgery, urinary calculi, and often an incidental finding. While CCA doesn't show these clinical features and often present hematuria or a visible bladder mass. A higher mitotic figures and prominent cellular atypia are ususally present microscopically in CCA [25, 31]. Immunohistochemically, elevated Ki-67 and p53 are helpful in differentiating the CCA from nephrogenic adenoma [24].

Treatment

Because of the rarity of CCA of the bladder, standard strategies for treating this neoplasm have not been established. No retrospective or prospective studies have been reported. Since most CCA tumors had muscular invasion or metastases at the initial diagnosis, the use of surgical resection combined with chemotherapy and radiotherapy is favorable [40]. Table 3 summerizes the treatments and outcomes of some CCA of the bladder cases in literatures published in English.

Surgical Resection

In all reviewed cases, initial treatment for primary clear cell carcinoma of the bladder was mainly surgical resection. All but 5 patients were initially treated with a surgical resection (89.1%, 41/46). The surgical resection therapy included transurethral resection (17 patients, 41.5%), total cystectomy (14 patients, 34.1%), radical surgery (5 patients, 12.2%), partial cystectomy (3 patients, 7.3%) and other surgical resection (2 patients, 4.9%; one underwent diverticulectomy, one underwent unspecific tumor resection). Of the 17 patients who underwent TUR-BT for their initial surgical treatment, 4 patients did not receive other therapies. One of these 4 patients presented no evidence of disease during 4-year follow-up period. Other patients underwent additional intravesical therapy, radical surgery, total cystectomy, chemotherapy and radiotherapy. Of the 14 patients who underwent total cystectomy for their initial surgical treatment, 9 patients did not receive other therapies. The longest follow-up period with no evidence of disease was 7 years.

Adding 2 patients with initial radiotherapy and subsequent surgery, there were totally 43 patients underwent surgical resection. At last follow-up (6-84 months), a total of 23 (53.5%) patients were alive with no evidence of disease, 9 (20.9%) patients were dead with disease, 8 (18.6%) patients were no data available and 3 (7.0%) patients were alive with disease.

Chemotherapy and Radiotherapy

It has been reported that chemotherapy was effective against clear cell adenocarcinomas of the gynecological organs [43]. One patient with Stage IV CCA of the bladder received chemotherapy and radiotherapy, and died with disease after 18 months [11]. Chemotherapy and radiotherapy have also been used as an adjuvant therapy for CCA.

Table 3. Treatment and outcomes of clear cell adenocarcinoma of the bladder in reported cases

References	Stage	Treatments	Follow-up(mo)	Outcomes
Dow, 1968 [2]	IV	RT,TC	12m	DWD
Skor, 1977 [6]	II	TC	24m	NED
Schultz, 1984 [7]	NA	TC	10m	NED
Young, 1985 [8]	NA	TUR	48m	NED
Chore, 1993 [9]	I	TC	NA	NA
Doria, 1996 [10]	NA	RS	15m	NED
Doria, 1996 [10]	NA	TC,CT,RT	84m	DWD
Drew, 1996 [11]	IV	CT,RT	18m	DWD
Drew, 1996 [11]	I	RS	12m	NED
Drew, 1996 [11]	I	TUR,RS	63m	A,P/P
Drew, 1996 [11]	I	TUR	30m	NED
Mai, 2000 [12]	NA	RS	NA	NA
Matsuoka, 2002 [13]	NA	TUR, RT	NA	NA
Matsuoka, 2002 [13]	NA	RT	24m	NED
Matsuoka, 2002 [13]	II	TC	9m	DWD
Matsuoka, 2002 [13]	NA	PC	36m	NED
Matsuoka, 2002 [13]	NA	TC	12m	DWD
Matsuoka, 2002 [13]	NA	TC	84m	NED
Matsuoka, 2002 [13]	NA	RT,TC	18m	NED
Matsuoka, 2002 [13]	NA	PC	60m	NED
Matsuoka, 2002 [13]	NA	TUR	NA	NA
Matsuoka, 2002 [13]	NA	TC	24m	NED
Matsuoka, 2002 [13]	NA	RS	NA	NA
Matsuoka, 2002 [13]	NA	TUR,RT	NA	NED
Matsuoka, 2002 [13]	NA	TUR,CT,TC	NA	NA
Matsuoka, 2002 [13]	NA	TC,RT	24m	DWD
Matsuoka, 2002 [13]	NA	TC	14m	NED
Matsuoka, 2002 [13]	NA	TUR,CT	25m	NED
Matsuoka, 2002 [13]	NA	TC,CT	18m	DWD
Matsuoka, 2002 [13]	NA	TC,CT	24m	DWD
Matsuoka, 2002 [13]	NA	RT	8m	DWD
Moinzadeh, 2003 [15]	NA	Diverticulectomy	12m	NED
Signori, 2003 [34]	T2	PC	6m	DWD
Kosem, 2005 [33]	NA	TUR,CT	18m	DWD
Kurosaka, 2005 [40]	T3a	TC,RT,CT	28m	NED
Lum, 2006 [32]	NA	Tumor resection	8m	NED
Adams, 2007 [31]	NA	TUR, RS	9m	NED
Sun, 2008 [25]	NA	TUR	NA	NA
Sun, 2008 [25]	NA	RS	10m	NED

Table 3. (Continued)

References	Stage	Treatments	Follow-up(mo)	Outcomes
Pena Alvarez, 2010 [41]	T2	TUR, RT, CT	24m	DWD
Rotellini, 2010 [30]	NA	TC	12m	NED
Sethi, 2011 [29]	NA	TUR, IVT, TC	6m	NED
Lu, 2012 [23]	T2a	TUR, IVT	12m	A,P/P
Szymanski, 2012 [28]	T3b	TUR, TC, CT	10m	NED
Abbas, 2013 [27]	T2	TUR, TC	NA	NA
Lah, 2013 [42]	NA	TUR,CT,RS	12m	NED

Abbreviations: A,P/P=alive with persistence or progression of disease; CT=chemotherapy; DWD=died with disease; IVT=intravesical therapy; NA=not available; NED=no evidence of disease; PC=partial cystectomy; RS=radical surgery; RT=radiotherapy; TC=total cystectomy.

Among 41 patients who received surgical resection as initial treatments, 13 patients underwent adjuvant chemotherapy (including cisplatin, doxorubicin or cyclophosphamide) and/or radiotherapy (40-60 Gy total) after surgery. One of them died of metastatic disease after 7 years [10]. One patient with advanced clear cell adenocarcinoma of the bladder (pT3a) has undergone radical surgery with adjuvant chemoradiothearapy, living without any evidence of recurrences during a 28-month observation [40]. 4 patients underwent radiotherapy as the initial treatment and two of them received total cystectomy later. Two of these four patients died with disease in 8 months and 1 year, respectively. The other two were alive with no evidence of disease in 18 months and 2 years, respectively [2, 13].

Intravesical Therapy

Although the intravesical therapy has been proven to be a valuable adjuvant therapy to TUR-BT for decreasing recurrence and progression of non-muscle-invasive bladder cancer [44], it seems ineffective for CCA of the bladder. Because of refusing any partial or radical cystectomy surgeries, one patient with CCA of the bladder underwent repeat intravesical therapy after TUR-BT but the tumor recurred in a short period of time [23].

Because some important information such as stages of CCA in these cases are not available, we are not able to do a meta-analysis for these data. Although some treatments or therapy regimens seem to have therapeutic efficacy on clear cell adenocarcinoma of the bladder, there is no sufficient evidence, such as retrospective or prospective studies with large case numbers, to confirm the efficacy of these treatments. However, on the basis of these reported cases, we suggest that immediate surgical intervention should be encouraged, if possible, to prevent further disease progression.

Prognosis

Based on the limited data, two patients with Stage IV disease died with disease within 2 years despite surgery and chemoradiotherapy, while patients with Stage I disease seems to have better prognosis [2, 11]. Because of the rarity of this disease, no other prognostic factors were identified. In general, it is more malignant than common urothelial carcinoma, but more cases and longer follow-up periods are required to elucidate these points. Lymph nodes and bone seem to be the most common metastatic sites for this disease [13, 33].

Conclusion

Primary clear cell adenocarcinoma of the bladder is a rare and aggressive tumor. Some demographic characteristics are distinct from those in patients with transitional cell carcinoma, but the clnical features are similar. The origin of this disease is still not clearly defined. Due to non-specific clnical features, diagnosis of CCA of the bladder is mainly based on histopathology. Immunohistochemistry of some markers also plays an important role in the diagnosis. Experiences are still accumulating in treating this disease. The standard treatment strategies have not been established because of the unavailability of large retrospective or prospective studies. Immediate surgical interventions are recommended to prevent further disease progression. Further investigations are needed to improve our knowledge in the diagnosis and treatment of this rare disease.

Acknowledgments

We are grateful to Dr. Qihui Chen, Department of Urology, The First Hospital of Jilin University, for permitting us to use two histopathological figures in this article.

References

[1] Eble JN, E.J., Seternhenn IA., World Health Organization Classification of Tumours. Pathology and Genetics, Tumours of the Urinary System and Male Genital organs. 2004, Lyon: IARC Press.

[2] Dow, J.A. and J.D. Young, Jr., Mesonephric adenocarcinoma of the bladder. *J Urol,* 1968. 100(4): p. 466-9.

[3] Ploeg, M., K.K. Aben, and L.A. Kiemeney, The present and future burden of urinary bladder cancer in the world. *World J Urol*, 2009. 27(3): p. 289-93.

[4] Fleshner, N.E., et al., The National Cancer Data Base report on bladder carcinoma. The American College of Surgeons Commission on Cancer and the American Cancer Society. *Cancer*, 1996. 78(7): p. 1505-13.

[5] Kantor, A.F., et al., Epidemiological characteristics of squamous cell carcinoma and adenocarcinoma of the bladder. *Cancer Res*, 1988. 48(13): p. 3853-5.

[6] Skor, A.B. and M.M. warren, Mesonephric adenocarcinoma of bladder. *Urology*, 1977. 10(1): p. 64-5.

[7] Schultz, R.E., et al., Mesonephric adenocarcinoma of the bladder. *J Urol,* 1984. 132(2): p. 263-5.

[8] Young, R.H. and R.E. Scully, Clear cell adenocarcinoma of the bladder and urethra. A report of three cases and review of the literature. *Am J Surg Pathol,* 1985. 9(11): p. 816-26.

[9] Chor, P.J., L.D. Gaum, and R.H. Young, Clear cell adenocarcinoma of the urinary bladder: report of a case of probable mullerian origin. *Mod Pathol,* 1993. 6(2): p. 225-8.

[10] Doria, M.I., Jr., et al., Cytologic features of clear cell carcinoma of the urethra and urinary bladder. *Diagn Cytopathol*, 1996. 14(2): p. 150-4.

[11] Drew, P.A., et al., The histogenesis of clear cell adenocarcinoma of the lower urinary tract. Case series and review of the literature. *Hum Pathol,* 1996. 27(3): p. 248-52.

[12] Mai, K.T., et al., Multicentric clear cell adenocarcinoma in the urinary bladder and the urethral diverticulum: evidence of origin of clear cell adenocarcinoma of the female lower urinary tract from Mullerian duct remnants. *Histopathology*, 2000. 36(4): p. 380-2.

[13] Matsuoka, Y., et al., Clear cell adenocarcinoma of the urinary bladder inducing acute renal failure. *Int J Urol*, 2002. 9(8): p. 467-9.

[14] Oliva, E., et al., Clear cell carcinoma of the urinary bladder: a report and comparison of four tumors of mullerian origin and nine of probable urothelial origin with discussion of histogenesis and diagnostic problems. *Am J Surg Pathol*, 2002. 26(2): p. 190-7.

[15] Moinzadeh, A., J. Latini, and K.J. Hamawy, Clear cell adenocarcinoma of the urinary bladder within a diverticulum. *Urology*, 2003. 62(1): p. 145.

[16] Oliva, E. and R.H. Young, Clear cell adenocarcinoma of the urethra: a clinicopathologic analysis of 19 cases. *Mod Pathol*, 1996. 9(5): p. 513-20.

[17] Peven, D.R. and D.F. Hidvegi, Clear-cell adenocarcinoma of the female urethra. *Acta Cytol,* 1985. 29(2): p. 142-6.

[18] Balat, O., et al., Malignant transformation in endometriosis of the urinary bladder: case report of clear cell adenocarcinoma. *Eur J Gynaecol Oncol,* 1996. 17(1): p. 13-6.

[19] Sung, M.T., et al., Histogenesis of clear cell adenocarcinoma in the urinary tract: evidence of urothelial origin. *Clin Cancer Res*, 2008. 14(7): p. 1947-55.

[20] Hartmann, A., et al., Molecular evidence for progression of nephrogenic metaplasia of the urinary bladder to clear cell adenocarcinoma. *Hum Pathol*, 2006. 37(1): p. 117-20.

[21] Gilcrease, M.Z., et al., Clear cell adenocarcinoma and nephrogenic adenoma of the urethra and urinary bladder: a histopathologic and immunohistochemical comparison. *Hum Pathol,* 1998. 29(12): p. 1451-6.

[22] Suttmann, H., et al., Mesonephroid adenocarcinoma arising from mesonephroid metaplasia of the urinary bladder. *Urology*, 2006. 67(4): p. 846 e7-8.

[23] Lu, J., et al., Primary clear cell adenocarcinoma of the bladder with recurrence: a case report and literature review. *World J Surg Oncol,* 2012. 10: p. 33.

[24] Herawi, M., et al., Clear cell adenocarcinoma of the bladder and urethra: cases diffusely mimicking nephrogenic adenoma. *Hum Pathol*, 2010. 41(4): p. 594-601.

[25] Sun, K., Y. Huan, and P.D. Unger, Clear cell adenocarcinoma of urinary bladder and urethra: another urinary tract lesion immunoreactive for P504S. *Arch Pathol Lab Med,* 2008. 132(9): p. 1417-22.

[26] Terada, T., An autopsy case of clear cell adenocarcinoma of the urinary bladder. Appl Immunohistochem *Mol Morphol*, 2013. 21(4): p. 371-5.

[27] Abbas, M., et al., Adenocarcinoma of the urinary bladder, mesonephroid type: a rare case. *Rare Tumors,* 2013. 5(1): p. e3.

[28] Szymanski, L.J., et al., A 50-year-old with gross hematuria. *Urology*, 2012. 80(3): p. 509-11.
[29] Sethi, S., S. Dhawan, and P. Chopra, Clear cell adenocarcinoma of urinary bladder: A case report and review. *Urol Ann*, 2011. 3(3): p. 151-4.
[30] Rotellini, M., et al., Clear cell carcinoma of the bladder in a patient with a earlier clear cell renal cell carcinoma: a case report with morphologic, immunohistochemical, and cytogenetical analysis. *Appl Immunohistochem Mol Morphol*, 2010. 18(4): p. 396-9.
[31] Adams, B., et al., A rare case of clear cell adenocarcinoma of the bladder with unique pathological features. *Am J Med Sci*, 2007. 333(1): p. 63-5.
[32] Lum, D., Clear cell carcinoma of the urinary bladder. *Pathology*, 2006. 38(4): p. 367-70.
[33] Kosem, M. and E. Sengul, Clear cell adenocarcinoma of the urinary bladder. *Scand J Urol Nephrol*, 2005. 39(1): p. 89-92.
[34] Signori, G., et al., Clear cell adenocarcinoma of the bladder in a male patient: clinicopathologic analysis of a case. *Urol Int*, 2003. 71(2): p. 228-30.
[35] Brimo, F., et al., Hepatocyte nuclear factor-1beta expression in clear cell adenocarcinomas of the bladder and urethra: diagnostic utility and implications for histogenesis. *Hum Pathol*, 2011. 42(11): p. 1613-9.
[36] Tong, G.X., et al., Expression of PAX8 in nephrogenic adenoma and clear cell adenocarcinoma of the lower urinary tract: evidence of related histogenesis? *Am J Surg Pathol*, 2008. 32(9): p. 1380-7.
[37] Whitworth, S.A., et al., Clear cell adenocarcinoma of the lower urinary tract: cytopathologic characteristics and differential diagnoses. *Cancer Cytopathol*, 2012. 120(5): p. 308-12.
[38] Orntoft, T.F. and H. Wolf, Molecular alterations in bladder cancer. *Urol Res*, 1998. 26(4): p. 223-33.
[39] Sandberg, A.A. and C.S. Berger, Review of chromosome studies in urological tumors. II. Cytogenetics and molecular genetics of bladder cancer. *J Urol*, 1994. 151(3): p. 545-60.
[40] Kurosaka, S., et al., Advanced clear-cell adenocarcinoma of the bladder successfully treated by radical surgery with adjuvant chemoradiotherapy. *Int J Clin Oncol*, 2005. 10(5): p. 362-5.
[41] Pena Alvarez, C., et al., Clear-cell adenocarcinoma of vesical origin: a case study of metastatic disease treated with chemotherapy. *Chemother Res Pract*, 2010. 2010: p. 426973.
[42] Lah, K., et al., Primary vesical clear cell adenocarcinoma arising in endometriosis: a rare case of mullerian origin. *Anticancer Res*, 2013. 33(2): p. 615-7.
[43] Ohta, I., et al., Cyclophosphamide and 5-fluorouracil act synergistically in ovarian clear cell adenocarcinoma cells. *Cancer Lett*, 2001. 162(1): p. 39-48.
[44] Braasch, M.R., A. Böhle, and M.A. O'Donnell, Intravesical Instillation Treatment of Non–muscle-invasive Bladder Cancer. *European Urology Supplements*, 2009. 8(7): p. 549-555.

In: Rare Diseases
Editors: Giorgio Di Giovanni and Pietro Marcoz

ISBN: 978-1-62948-525-6

Chapter VIII

Eosinophilic Pancreatitis

Sanem Guler, Sertac Cimen, Frank MacDonald, Scott Hurton and Michele Molinari*

Dalhousie University, Department of Surgery, Victoria General Hospital, Victoria Building, Halifax, Nova Scotia, Canada

Abstract

Eosinophilic pancreatitis (EP) is an extremely rare clinical entity. So far, only 26 cases of EP have been reported in the medical literature. Most of the patients with EP are also affected by eosinophilic gastroenteritis (EG) (88%) or idiopathic hypereosinophilic syndrome (HIS). Hypersensitivity reactions and milk allergy are considered common etiological factors for both EP and EG. For the majority of patients, the diagnosis can be challenging because of the wide array of non-specific symptoms such as recurrent abdominal pain, diarrhea and weight loss. The main treatment of EP is the use of steroids and the prognosis is usually favorable with resolution of the symptoms and histopahological findings. Endoscopy is often used to obtain biopsies and to insert temporary stents in the biliary or pancreatic ducts in patients who present with jaundice or pancreatic duct obstruction.

Introduction

Eosinophilic pancreatitis (EP) is an uncommon clinical entity [1] and to date, only 26 cases have been reported. In all but one, EP was in association with eosinophilic gastroenteritis (EG) or idiopathic hypereosinophilic syndrome (IHS) [1-3]. Only 1 case of 'isolated' EP has been observed in a newborn of a diabetic mother [4]. The diagnosis was made only after the newborn died and an autopsy was performed. Approximately, 85% of the

* Corresponding author: Michele Molinari: Telephone: 902-473-7624. Fax: 902-473-7639. Email: michele.molinari@cdha.nshealth.ca.

patients with EP have concurrent EG (22 of 26 cases) and the remaining are affected by IHS (3 of 26 cases). In this book chapter, 'EP associated with EG' and 'EP associated with IHS' will be discussed as two separate entities although their clinical presentation and management may overlap.

Clinical Presentation of Eosinophilic Pancreatitis (EP)

The clinical presentation of patients with EP is similar to patients affected by other causes of pancreatitis. The initial symptoms are vague abdominal pain, anorexia and weight loss, steatorrhea and, in some cases, obstructive jaundice due to occlusion of the intra-pancreatic bile duct [5, 1, 6-9]. In patients with involvement of the pancreatic body and tail, the most frequent clinical presentation is the presence of persistent epigastrium and mid-abdominal pain associated with radiological findings mimicking pancreatic cancer [2]. Less frequently, these patients may present with pseudocysts and stenosis of the main pancreatic duct with proximal ductal dilatation [9, 10]. Patients with EP associated with EG may present with early diarrhea and recurrent intestinal obstructions due to edema of the intestinal wall. On the other hand, patients with EP and IHS often present with allergic-type symptoms and thickening of the serosa of the intra-thoracic or intra-abdominal organs with various degrees of hydrothorax or ascites [1, 7, 9, 11].

Eosinophilic Pancreatitis Associated with Eosinophilic Gastroenteritis

Eosinophilic gastroenteritis (EG) is an inflammatory condition that is characterized by focal or diffuse eosinophilic infiltration of the gastrointestinal tract [1]. Similar to Crohn's disease, EG can involve any part of the intestine from the esophagus to the rectum [11]. It usually presents in the third to fifth decade, with a male to female ratio of 3:2 [12]. It was first described in 1937 by Kaijser, who reported two patients with an allergy to neoarsphenamine, a derivative of arsphenamine once used to treat syphilis and yaws [11, 12]. Since then, more than 300 cases of EG have been reported [13].

Etiology of Eosinophilic Gastroenteritis (EG)

The actual cause of EG is unknown but it is suspected that the majority of cases are due to an allergic reaction [11] as a personal or family history of food allergies and atopic disorders are present in 50-70% of cases [5, 14]. In general, males are more frequently affected than females [12].

Clinical Presentation of Eosinophilic Gastroenteritis (EG)

The following symptoms and findings are common in patients affected by EG [12]:

- Nausea, vomiting, diarrhea, bloating, diffuse abdominal pain, anemia and weight loss
- Eosinophilic infiltration of the intestinal wall in biopsies obtained during endoscopic investigations
- Absence of any recognizable parasitic infection

All patients with EG develop eosinophilic infiltration in the wall of the gastrointestinal tract involved [11]. Although any part of the intestine can be affected, it is more frequent in the stomach and in the small intestine and dignosis can be done by upper endoscopy and biopsy. Symptoms of EG depend on the location and depth of the eosinophilic infiltration [11, 13]. Although most of the patients have peripheral eosinophilia along with elevated serum IgE levels [12], peripheral eosinophil count is not a sensitive test since it is normal in 23% of patients and can be elevated in patients with other forms of pancreatitis [15].

Types of Eosinophilic Gastroenteritis (EG)

Klein et al. [16] classified EG into three groups based on the depth of the eosinophilic infiltration in the gut. The first class is the mucosal disease that is the most frequent form and it may be associated with anemia, protein losing enteropathy and malabsorption. The second largest group is made by patients affected by muscle layer infiltration who typically present with intermittent intestinal obstructions. The least common form of EG is the serosal disease. This group of patients usually has higher eosinophil counts in the peripheral blood than the patients with the other types of EG [17].

Eosinophilic Gastroenteritis (EG) with Concomitant Eosinophilic Pancreatitis (EP)

Twenty-two cases of 'EP with EG' have been reported so far in the medical literature [2, 5-8, 10, 12-14, 17-20]. EP can be seen at any age, however, it is more common in the 4th decade of life or in older patients (10 of 22 patients) (Table 1). Males and females are equally affected and the overall estimated life-time risk of developing pancreatitis in individuals affected by EG is in the order of 1-2% [13]. The most common symptoms of 'EG with EP' are abdominal pain, nausea, vomiting, recurrent abdominal distention and persistent diarrhea [13, 21]. One third of the cases were afflicted by significant weight loss due to malabsorption. Eight of the 22 reported cases presented with obstructive jaundice [6-9, 18, 19, 22].

Several factors seem to be responsible for EG and EP. Food allergy and atopy are the most consistent [5, 6, 9, 12, 13, 17, 19, 21].

Table 1. Demographics, clinical presentation and treatment modalities of EP patients associated with EG

Ref	Year of publication (Country)	N. of Patient	Gender (Age)	Clinical Presentation	History of Allergy	Treatment
[18]	1973) (Spain)	1	M (40)	Epigastric pain, nausea, vomiting, jaundice	N.A.	Billroth I subtotal gastrectomy, choledochotomy, duodenotomy. tube insertion
[23]	1975 (United States)	1	M (39)	Abdominal pain, nausea, vomiting, chills, fever	Negative	Radical pancreaticoduodenectomy, cholecystectomy, antrectomy, vagotomy
[21]	1979 (United States)	1	M (54)	Epigastric pain, nausea	Penicillin	Cystogastrostomy
[2]	1990 (France)	1	M (21)	Epigastric pain	Negative	En bloc resection of the tail of the pancreas, spleen, splenic flexure of the colon, and lymph nodes
[6]	1998 (France)	2	M (64)	Weight loss, jaundice	N.A.	Antrectomy, gastrojejunal anastomosis, along with a biliary digestive by-pass
[6]	1998 (France)	2	M (18)	Epigastric pain, jaundice, weight loss	Asthma	Pancreaticoduodenectomy
[20]	1997 (Japan)	1	M (27)	Nausea, vomiting, diarrhea, abdominal pain	Negative	Steroid
[1]	2000 (United States)	1	M (36)	Epigastric pain, nausea, anorexia, weight loss, fatigue	Negative	Pylorus-sparing pancreaticoduodenectomy
[14]	2002 (United States)	1	F (59)	Abdominal pain, nausea, vomiting, weight loss	Negative	ERCP-sphincterotomy
[9]	2003 (United States)	3	M (60)	Abdominal pain, jaundice	Asthma	Total pancreatectomy
[9]	2003 (United States)	3	F (36)	Abdominal pain	N.A.	Pancreaticoduodenectomy
[9]	2003 (United States)	3	M (41)	Abdominal pain	N.A.	Pancreaticoduodenectomy
[17]	2004 (United States)	1	F (30)	Nausea, vomiting, diarrhea, abdominal pain, weight loss	Rhinitis	Steroid
[7]	2006 (Turkey)	1	M (14)	Vomiting, abdominal pain, jaundice	N.A.	Laparotomy -pancreatic biopsy - Methylprednisolone
[8]	2006 (United States)	1	M (40)	Epigastric pain, nausea, vomiting, jaundice	N.A.	Pancreaticoduodenectomy
[13]	2006 (Denmark)	1	F (35)	Abdominal pain, vomiting	Horse and cat	Billroth 2 with gastrojejunostomy and enteroanastomosis
[10]	2007 (India)	1	F (38)	Abdominal distension, fever, weakness	N.A.	Surgical drainage of pseudocyst, cholecystectomy + Steroid
[12]	2009 (United States)	2	F (60)	Abdominal pain, nausea, vomiting, diarrhea	Asthma	Steroid
[12]	2009 (United States)	2	M (43)	Abdominal pain, nausea, vomiting, diarrhea, weight loss	Asthma	Steroid, sodium chromoglycate
[19]	2012 (Turkey)	1	F (17)	Nausea, abdominal pain, weight loss, jaundice	Cow milk allergy	Laparoscopic full thickness biopsy; Steroid
[5]	2012 (Japan)	1	M (28)	Nausea, vomiting, epigastric pain	Cow milk allergy	Steroid, epinastine hydrochloride, montelucast sodium
[22]	2003 (Korea)	1	F(65)	Epigastric pain, jaundice, pruritis, weight loss	N.A.	Steroid

Legends: N.A.= Not available.

When an allergen is clearly identified, elimination of the offending substance can lead to complete convalescence. In fact, Caglar [19] and Suzuki [5] observed complete resolution of EG and EP in patients affected by cow milk allergy (Table 1). Allergic rhinitis, asthma and inflammatory disorders with atopy-like pathophysiology have also been identified as risk factors by several other groups [6, 9, 12, 13, 17]. On the other hand, data regarding the association of 'EP with EG' and history of smoking and alcohol abuse remains inconclusive as only 3 of 22 (14%) previously reported 'EP with EG' patients had a history of alcohol consumption [1, 21, 22].

Pathogenesis of Eosinophilic Pancreatitis (EP)

The pathogenesis of EP depends either by direct eosinophilic infiltration of the pancreatic parenchyma or by the stenosis of the papilla of Vater due to eosinophilic infiltration of the duodenum [19]. Recognition of which mechanism is responsible for the cause of pancreatitis may play an important role. In fact, endoscopic stenting of the pancreatic duct can be indicated in patients with pancreatitis due to inflammation of the papilla of Vater [19].

Table 2. Endoscopy and laboratory findings of patients with EP associated with EG

Ref	Endoscopy/ Biopsy	Serum Amylase (IU/L)	Serum Lipase (IU/L)	Eosinophilia	Elevated Serum IgE level
[18]	Normal	1600	NA	Positive	N.A.
[23]	Upper GIS series: lesion narrowing the second portion of duodenum	N.A.	NA	Negative	N.A.
[21]	Normal (Barium study)	786	NA	Positive	Positive
[2]	Duodenal ulcer (8mm) Biopsy: Non-specific	358	1013	Positive	N.A.
[6]	Normal- no biopsy	Normal	Normal	Negative	Negative
[6]	NA (presumed diagnosis of Neuroendocrine pancreatic tumor)	135	Normal	Positive	Positive
[20]	Swelling of the papilla. Biopsy: Eosinophilic infiltration	2340	477	Positive	Positive
[1]	ERCP/ Stricture	1505	4828	Negative	N.A.
[14]	Eosinophils in the lamina propria, mucosa of duodenum and stomach	392	N.A.	Positive	N.A.
[9]	ERCP/ biliary strictures	N.A.	N.A.	Positive	N.A.
[9]	ERCP/ biliary strictures	N.A.	N.A.	Positive	N.A.
[9]	NA	N.A.	N.A.	Positive	N.A.
[17]	Gastritis and duodenitis, eosinophils in submucosa	94	1057	Positive	N.A.
[7]	Duodenum and ampulla of Vater biopsy Eosinophils in lamina propria	593	N.A.	Positive	Positive
[8]	Duodenal compression and ampullitis, eosinophilic infiltrate in lamina propria	N.A.	2100	Positive	N.A.
[13]	Erosive duodenitis, eosinophils in lamina propria	1605	Normal	Positive	N.A.
[10]	A localized bulge on the body of the stomach on the greater curvature	450	276	Positive	Positive
[12]	Distal esophagitis, antral gastritis, duodenitis Biopsy: Eosinophilic infiltration	375	1115	Positive	Negative
[12]	Esophagitis, multiple antral erosions, ulcerated nodules in the duodenal bulb, Biopsy: Eosinophilic infiltration	471	1785	Positive	Positive
[19]	Thickened gastric folds, edematous and erosive bulbus. Biopsy: Eosinophilic infiltrate	764	1037	Positive	Positive
[5]	Mild esophagitis, erosive gastritis, and duodenitis. Biopsy: Eosinophilic infiltrate	Normal	202	Positive	Negative
[22]	ERCP/ biliary strictures	258	416	Negative	Positive

Legends: N.A.= Not available.

Laboratory Findings

In 82% of patients affected by EP, peripheral eosinophil count is elevated (Table 2). In comparison to patients with isolated EG, patients with concomitant EP and EG are more often diagnosed with peripheral eosinophilia that seems to be due to the more extensive disease. Elevation of serum amylase and lipase are seen in 82% and 59% of the cases respectively [1, 2, 5, 7, 8, 10, 12-14, 17-22].

Gastrointestinal Studies

Most of the patients with EP and EG present with non-specific gastrointestinal symptoms and undergo endoscopic investigations. Among all the 20 published cases where endoscopic studies were performed, 15 patients displayed involvement of the stomach, duodenum or ampulla of Vater (Table 2).

Endoscopic biopsy of 9 of these cases revealed eosinophilic infiltration of the lamina propria while 1 of them disclosed involvement of the submucosal layer [7, 8, 12-14, 17, 19, 20]. The classical endoscopic findings of EG include an erythematous, friable and nodular mucosal layer with occasional ulcerative changes (Figure 1) [19]. However, a normal endoscopic study does not totally exclude the diagnosis of EG since patients might be affected by skip lesions [11] (Table 2).

Serosal disease is more difficult to diagnose as there are no studies that are very sensitive or specific for this condition. Interestingly enough, among all 5 reported patients who had serosal involvement and who had ascites on abdominal ultrasound, analysis of the ascitic fluid revealed elevation of the eosinophilic count [8, 10, 13, 17, 19].

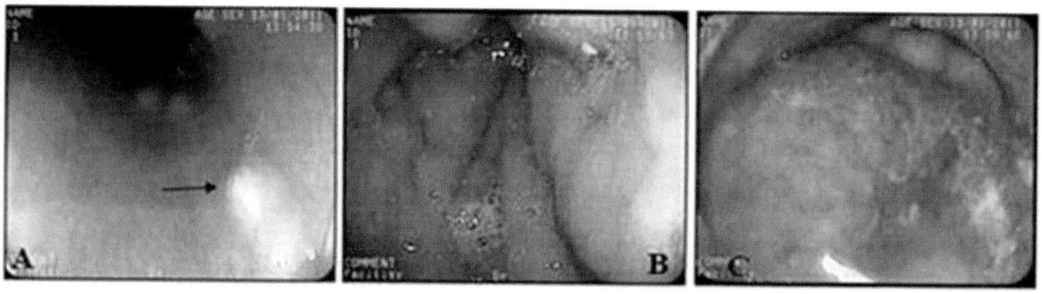

Figure 1. Endoscopic appearance of eosinophilic gastroenteritis. Endoscopic view of a Turkish patient affected by abdominal pain and weight loss. During upper endoscopy, pearly white colored thin mucosal nodularities were seen in the esophagus (A; black arrow). In the body of the stomach, the patient had erythematous, hypertrophic gastric folds (B) and a prominent scalloping covered by edematous, erythematous and erosive mucosa in the bulbus (C) (Courtesy of Caglar et al.) (A case of eosinophilic gastroenteritis mimicking gastric lymphoma associated with pancreatitis due to duodenal involvement, Istanbul, Turkey, 2012).

Conclusion

Diagnosis of 'EP with concomitant EG' should be in the differential diagnosis of patients with gastrointestinal symptoms and pancreatitis. Elevated levels of serum IgE, amylase and lipase along with eosinophilia in the absence of parasitic infestations are supportive findings. Upper endoscopy can be very useful as 85% of patients will have visible abnormalities of the mucosa or histopathological findings consistent with eosinophilic infiltration in their biopsies.

Eosinophilic Pancreatitis (EP) Associated with Idiopathic Hypereosinophilic Syndrome (HIS)

IHS but not EG has been diagnosed in 3 of the 26 cases of EP reported in the literature so far. IHS is a rare leukoproliferative disorder characterized by idiopathic elevation of the number of eosinophils in the peripheral blood with some degree of organ damage [24].

In this condition, eosinophils tend to infiltrate several solid organs where they de-granulate and release cytotoxic proteins and peroxidases. If the process is not stopped, the damage to the target organ can become irreversible [25]. These patients might present with a variety of symptoms that depend on which organs are involved.

In 1975, Chusid et al. [26] described the diagnostic parameters of IHS:

- Presence of greater than 1500/μl eosinophils in peripheral blood of patients for period of time equal or longer than 6 months
- No other reason for the eosinophilia and no evidence of clonality
- Signs and symptoms of organ dysfunction

The main aim for the treatment of these patients is the reduction of their eosinophilia as it may slow down the progression of organ damage.

Oral and intraveneous steroids, hydroxyurea, interferon alpha and imatinib have been used for these patients [27]. In more recent years, Mepolizumab (SB-240563), a humanized mouse anti-human IL-5 monoclonal antibody has been proven to be effective and safe in the treatment of patients with IHS [27].

Eosinophilic Pancreatitis with Idiopathic Hypereosinophilic Syndrome

Only three cases of patients affected by EP in association with IHS have been reported so far. The clinical presentations of these patients are summarized in Table 3. Abdominal pain was the chief complaint of all of them [28-30]. One of the cases had a markedly elevated serum level of the tumor marker Ca 19-9 and underwent a duodenopancreatectomy (Whipple procedure) for a suspected pancreatic cancer of the uncinate process [28] (Table 3). The two other patients received medical treatment instead [29, 30].

Table 3. Gender, clinical presentation, laboratory findings and treatment modalities of EP patients associated with HIS

Ref	Gender (Age)	Clinical Presentation	Eosinophilia	Elevated Serum IgE level	Allergy	Amylase	Lipase	Treatment	Radiological Tests / Endoscopic Findings
[28]	F (74)	Abdominal pain, jaundice, itching, weight loss, fever	Positive	N.A.	N.A.	High	High	Pancreaticoduodenectomy	Mass at the head of pancreas on abdominal CT
[29]	F (37)	Abdominal pain	Positive	Positive	Mite allergy	1200	1030	Cromolyn	Normal
[30]	F (71)	Weight loss, epigastric pain, pruritis, diarrhea	Positive	Normal	N.A.	N.A.	High	Steroids	CT: Enlarged pancreas Endoscopic Biopsy (Eosinophilic infiltration)

Legends: N.A.= Not available.

Diagnosis of Eosinophilic Pancreatitis with Idiopathic Hypereosinophilic Syndrome

High peripheral eosinophil count, elevated serum IgE, amylase and lipase levels are prominent laboratory findings of EP as previously mentioned.

Additionally, diagnosis of EP may requires multiple imaging studies including endoscopy, endoscopic ultrasound (EUS), computerized tomography (CT), endoscopic retrograde cholangiopancreatography (ERCP) and magnetic resonance cholangiopancreatography (MRCP). The most common endoscopic findings of 'EP with EG' are thickening of the antral gastric mucosa and ulcer in the duodenal bulb [19]. Edema of the papillary region of the duodenum may be the reason for the concurrent obstructive jaundice. However, these findings are non-specific since they can also be present in Crohn's disease and lymphoma [19]. Although any part of the gastrointestinal tract can be involved, esophagus and colon are the least likely involved sites [5]. Colonoscopic biopsy revealed eosinophilic colitis in only 1 case reported in the literature [12]. However, the prevalence of esophageal involvement has increased recently [12, 25]. In most of the cases with positive endoscopic findings, 3 weeks of steroid treatment was sufficient for endoscopy-proven remission of the disease [11]. EUS can help in diagnosis especially when combined with fine needle aspiration (EUS-FNA). Suspicious pancreatic lesions can be sampled by this method with very low complication rates [25]. This strategy may prevent unnecessary pancreatic surgeries in patients presenting with resectable pancreatic mass and eosinophilia [6]. CT scan can detect suspicious pancreatic masses and pseudocysts. Among 26 reported EP cases, 6 had a pancreatic mass while 5 had pseudocysts revealed by CT scan [1, 3, 6, 7, 9, 10, 21, 22, 28]. Enlargement of the pancreatic head and pancreatic duct dilation are other potential CT scan findings of EP patients. EUS and EUS-FNA can be used to further characterize the CT scan findings [1]. ERCP had a significant role in diagnostic work-up of EP, especially before the introduction of MRCP. Focal areas of stricture in the pancreatic duct consist the most striking ERCP finding [1, 2, 9]. However, this finding is not specific, as it may also be present in pancreatic malignancies. There is 1 case in the literature with an ERCP finding of complete pancreatic duct narrowing probably due to extensive eosinophilic infiltration of the pancreas parenchyma [6]. Complete narrowing of the pancreatic duct can be seen in autoimmune pancreatitis as well. Another indication of ERCP is stent insertion and/or sphincterotomy in EP patients with biliary obstruction and jaundice [14, 30]. After its introduction, MRCP has become the preferred method for investigation of pancreatic and biliary tree in EP patients without obstructive jaundice [31]. Ryan et al. [23] reported a case in which selective arteriography of the pancreas was included in the diagnostic workup. Pancreatic arteriography was performed in this case by selective celiac axis and superior mesenteric artery catheterization. The arterial supply of the head of the pancreas and the pancreatic mass was normal. This case-which is unique in the literature with selective arteriographic imaging of the pancreas-showed that in the setting of EP arterial blood supply to the pancreatic mass is not increased in contrast to malignant pancreatic tumors [23].

Pathological Features

The most prominent histopathological feature of EP is increased eosinophil count (equal or more than 20/high power field) in the pancreatic parenchyma [7] with associated peripheral eosinophilia in the absence of an identifiable cause [5] (Figure 2).

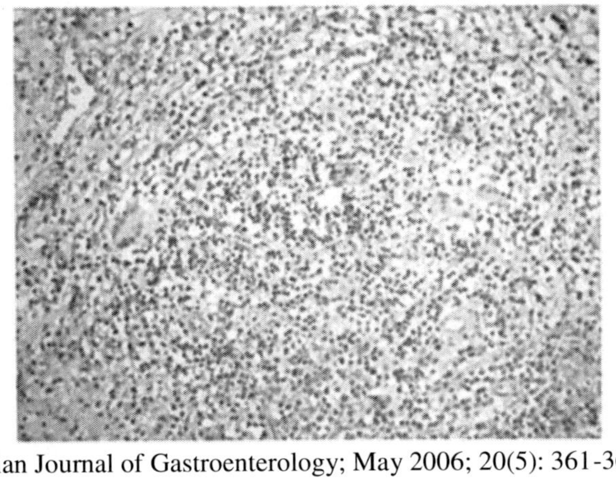

(Courtesy of the Canadian Journal of Gastroenterology; May 2006; 20(5): 361-364).

Figure 2. Histopathological features of eosinophilic pancreatitis. It is noticeable the signifycant eosinophilic infiltrate in the pancreatic parenchyma.

Two different histological patterns have been described [9]. In the first, the entire pancreas is enlarged and fibrotic, there is diffuse eosinophilic infiltrate within the septae and around the pancreatic ducts and acini. Additionally, eosinophilic phlebitis or arteritis may be present. The second pattern is characterized by pancreatic pseudocysts consisting of dense fibrosis and intense eosinophilic infiltrate that spares the more distal pancreatic parenchyma.

Although distinctive histopathological features of these patterns are known, the pathogenic mechanism of each pattern remains unknown.

Differential Diagnosis

The differential diagnosis of EP from other forms of pancreatitis may be very difficult [13]. Its association with either EG or IHS is in itself a diagnostic challenge since patients have symptoms and signs due to these rare conditions [13]. Parasitic infestation, pancreatic carcinoma, acute/chronic pancreatitis, carcinoma of the duodenum, peptic ulcer disease, regional enteritis, post-surgical stricture and gallstone disease must all be included in the differential diagnosis [7, 19].

Treatment of Eosinophilic Pancreatitis (EP)

Treatment of EP should be patient-tailored [28]. The severity of the symptoms and the degree of the disease must be considered when selecting treatment modalities. Medical treatment should be started as soon as the diagnosis is confirmed [12]. Steroids are the mainstay of the medical therapy for patients with 'EP in the presence of EG' [19]. Steroid therapy, particularly, oral prednisolone, has been the cornerstone of the treatment, with doses of up to 40mg/day [17]. Improvement is typically noted within the first two to three weeks, although prolonged courses of treatment may be necessary in some cases. Most of the patients have no recurrence [5]. In case where recurrence is seen, patients might require long-term steroid treatment [5]. Because of the rarity of this condition, the optimal duration of steroids is still unknown. Various steroid sparing agents such as sodium cromoglycate (mast cell membrane stabilizer), ketotifen (antihistamine) and montelukast (a selective, competitive leukotriene receptor antagonist) have been used with variable success rates [2, 5, 29].

Eosinophilic infiltration of the pancreas resembling pancreatic mass in CT scan or EUS may suggest pancreatic carcinoma (Table 1, 3). These patients may also have the additional characteristic features of pancreatic cancer such as obstructive jaundice and weight loss. Altogether, these clinical features and the rarity of EP may lead to the provisional diagnosis of pancreas carcinoma and subsequent surgical resection. After surgery, there is high risk of fistula formation due to impaired healing of duodenal tissue as a result of eosinophilic infiltration [13, 18]. Surgical intervention should be avoided if diagnosis of EP is made with reasonable confidence. Stent insertion or sphincterotomy may be recommended in patients with biliary obstruction. Although 'EP with EG' may relapse after treatment, they respond to medical therapy and the expected overall prognosis is favorable [19].

Conclusion

EP is a rare clinical entity [1]. The diagnosis of EP should be entertained when no other causes of pancreatitis are identified, especially in patients with peripheral eosinophilia and without identifiable infections [19]. Clinicians should keep in mind that there is a strong association between EP and EG or IHS because the demonstration of eosinophilic infiltration in tissues obtained during endoscopic biopsy can be useful to support the diagnosis of EP [18]. The main treatment of EP is the use of steroids and the prognosis is usually favorable with resolution of the symptoms and histopahological findings. Endoscopy is often used to obtain biopsies and to insert temporary stents in the biliary or pancreatic ducts in patients who present with jaundice or pancreatic duct obstruction.

References

[1] Euscher E, Vaswani K, Frankel W: Eosinophilic pancreatitis: a rare entity that can mimic a pancreatic neoplasm. *Ann. Diagn. Pathol.* 2000; 4:379-85.

[2] Bastid C, Sahel J, Choux R, Payan MJ, Sarles H: Eosinophilic pancreatitis: report of a case. *Pancreas* 1990; 5:104-7.

[3] Chandrasekar TS, Goenka MK, Lawrence R, Gokul BJ, Murugesh M, Menachery J: An unusual case of ascites. *Indian J. Gastroenterol.* 2012; 31:203-7.

[4] Barresi G, Inferrera C, De Luca F: Eosinophilic pancreatitis in the newborn infant of a diabetic mother. *Virchows Arch. A Pathol. Anat. Histol.* 1978; 380:341-8.

[5] Suzuki S, Homma T, Kurokawa M, et al.: Eosinophilic gastroenteritis due to cow's milk allergy presenting with acute pancreatitis. *Int. Arch. Allergy Immunol.* 2012; 158 Suppl 1:75-82.

[6] Barthet M, Hastier P, Buckley MJ, et al.: Eosinophilic pancreatitis mimicking pancreatic neoplasia: EUS and ERCP findings--is nonsurgical diagnosis possible? *Pancreas* 1998; 17:419-22.

[7] Cay A, Imamoglu M, Cobanoglu U: Eosinophilic pancreatitis mimicking pancreatic neoplasia. *Can. J. Gastroenterol.* 2006;20:361-4.

[8] Stevens T, Mackey R, Falk GW, Bennett A, Henderson JM: Eosinophilic pancreatitis presenting as a pancreatic mass with obstructive jaundice. *Gastrointest. Endosc.* 2006; 63:525-7.

[9] Abraham SC, Leach S, Yeo CJ, et al.: Eosinophilic pancreatitis and increased eosinophils in the pancreas. *Am. J. Surg. Pathol.* 2003; 27:334-42.

[10] Rakesh K, Banerjee R, Gupta R, et al.: Eosinophilic pancreatitis with pseudocyst. *Indian J. Gastroenterol.* 2007; 26:136-7.

[11] Talley NJ, Shorter RG, Phillips SF, Zinsmeister AR: Eosinophilic gastroenteritis: a clinicopathological study of patients with disease of the mucosa, muscle layer, and subserosal tissues. *Gut* 1990; 31:54-8.

[12] Sheikh RA, Prindiville TP, Pecha RE, Ruebner BH: Unusual presentations of eosinophilic gastroenteritis: case series and review of literature. *World J. Gastroenterol.* 2009; 15:2156-61.

[13] Lyngbaek S, Adamsen S, Aru A, Bergenfeldt M: Recurrent acute pancreatitis due to eosinophilic gastroenteritis. Case report and literature review. *JOP* 2006;7:211-7.

[14] Polyak S, Smith TA, Mertz H: Eosinophilic gastroenteritis causing pancreatitis and pancreaticobiliary ductal dilation. *Dig. Dis. Sci.* 2002; 47:1091-5.

[15] Tokoo M, Oguchi H, Kawa S, Homma T, Nagata A: Eosinophilia associated with chronic pancreatitis: an analysis of 122 patients with definite chronic pancreatitis. *Am. J. Gastroenterol.* 1992; 87:455-60.

[16] Klein NC, Hargrove RL, Sleisenger MH, Jeffries GH: Eosinophilic gastroenteritis. *Medicine* (Baltimore) 1970; 49:299-319.

[17] Le Connie D, Nguyen H: Eosinophilic gastroenteritis, ascites, and pancreatitis: a case report and review of the literature. *South Med. J.* 2004; 97:905-6.

[18] Vazquez Rodriguez JJ, Soleto Saez E, Sanchez Vega J, Lopez Serrano MC, Cerdan Vallejo A: Pancreatitis and eosinophilic gastroenteritis. *Int. Surg.* 1973; 58:415-9.

[19] Caglar E, Karismaz K, Dobrucali A: A case of eosinophilic gastroenteritis mimicking gastric lymphoma associated with pancreatitis due to duodenal involvement. *Turk. J. Gastroenterol.* 2012; 23:585-9.

[20] Maeshima A, Murakami H, Sadakata H, et al.: Eosinophilic gastroenteritis presenting with acute pancreatitis. *J. Med.* 1997; 28:265-72.

[21] Hashimoto F: Transient eosinophilia associated with pancreatitis and pseudocyst formation. *Arch. Intern. Med.* 1980; 140:1099-100.

[22] Song JW, Kim MH, Seo WJ, et al.: [A case of eosinophilic pancreatitis]. *Korean J. Gastroenterol.* 2003; 42:444-50.

[23] Ryan KG: Eosinophilic infiltration of duodenum and pancreatic head: report of a case studied arteriographically. *Surgery* 1975; 77:321-4.

[24] Helbig G, Wisniewska-Piaty K, Francuz T, Dziaczkowska-Suszek J, Kyrcz-Krzemien S: Diversity of clinical manifestations and response to corticosteroids for idiopathic hypereosinophilic syndrome: retrospective study in 33 patients. *Leuk Lymphoma* 2013; 54:807-11.

[25] Agarwal B, Krishna NB, Labundy JL, Safdar R, Akduman EI: EUS and/or EUS-guided FNA in patients with CT and/or magnetic resonance imaging findings of enlarged pancreatic head or dilated pancreatic duct with or without a dilated common bile duct. *Gastrointest. Endosc.* 2008; 68:237-42; quiz 334, 5.

[26] Chusid MJ, Dale DC, West BC, Wolff SM: The hypereosinophilic syndrome: analysis of fourteen cases with review of the literature. *Medicine* (Baltimore) 1975; 54:1-27.

[27] Cogan E, Roufosse F: Clinical management of the hypereosinophilic syndromes. *Expert Rev. Hematol.* 2012; 5:275-89; quiz 90.

[28] Bellaiche G, Fontaine H, Choudat L, Lusina D, Ley G, Slama JL: [Pancreatic involvement, ascites and diarrhea in idiopathic hypereosinophilic syndrome]. *Gastroenterol. Clin. Biol.* 1997; 21:519-22.

[29] Roy-Peaud F, Paccalin M, Le Moal G, Landron C, Roblot P, Becq-Giraudon B: [Eosinophilic pancreatitis]. *Presse Med.* 2002; 31:25.

[30] Atig A, Ben Jazia E, Alaoua A, et al.: Acute pancreatitis due to idiopathic hypereosinophilic syndrome: a case report. *Acta Endosc.* 2011; 41:26-8.

[31] Krishna NB, Mehra M, Reddy AV, Agarwal B: EUS/EUS-FNA for suspected pancreatic cancer: influence of chronic pancreatitis and clinical presentation with or without obstructive jaundice on performance characteristics. *Gastrointest. Endosc.* 2009; 70:70-9.

In: Rare Diseases
Editors: Giorgio Di Giovanni and Pietro Marcoz
ISBN: 978-1-62948-525-6

Chapter IX

Non-Traumatic Splenic Rupture: An Enigma in Emergency

Jitendra Kumar Kushwaha[1,*], Abhinav Arun Sonkar[1], Akshay Anand[1] and Suyash Singh[1]
[1]Department of Surgery, King George's Medical University, Lucknow, UP, India

Abstract

Splenic rupture is a rare cause of abdominal pain and carries a high mortality rate. While the most common cause is trauma, it may occur due to the complications of infectious, neoplastic and hematologic diseases. Patients usually suffer from acute abdominal pain in the left upper quadrant, nausea, vomiting, and dizziness. Ultrasonography is important for diagnosis and abdominal computed tomography is important especially for staging the splenic rupture. For the treatment, either splenectomy or follow-up (especially for low-grade splenic ruptures) can be done.

The therapy of choice can vary between patients depending on grade of splenic rupture, hemodynamic instability, availability of endovascular treatment and preference of the treating physician.

Treatment should be focused on preserving splenic tissue. Non-traumatic rupture of the spleen must be considered by physicians in patients presenting with acute abdominal pain even without evident history of trauma, since early recognition and treatment can prevent serious morbidity and mortality. It has the same clinical picture as traumatic rupture of the spleen but the presentation can be vague and easily missed due to the absence of trauma or other predisposing factors. Increased awareness of this condition would enhance early diagnosis and effective treatment.

* E-mail: dr.jkkushwaha@gmail.com.

Introduction

Spleen plays an important role in the host defense against number of capsulated and intravascular microorganisms including Plasmodium. Traumatic splenic rupture is common while non-traumatic splenic rupture may occur in 0.1% - 0.5% of patients with no associated trauma [1]. The first cases of spontaneous splenic rupture were reported by Rokitansky [2] in 1861 and Atkinson [3] in 1874. Rupture of the spleen is a potentially life threatening complication usually occurring after blunt abdominal trauma with a frequency up to 40% [4]. Unlike traumatic splenic rupture spontaneous non-traumatic splenic rupture is extremely rare. The term spontaneous splenic rupture is poorly defined [5].

Characterization of Non-Traumatic Splenic Trauma

Non-traumatic rupture of the spleen due to known cause is extremely rare [6-9]. Orloff and Peksin [10], identified four criteria for the diagnosis of non traumatic spontaneous splenic rupture: (1) there should be no history of trauma or unusual activity what so ever; (2) there should be no evidence of disease in other organs that are known to affect the spleen directly or indirectly; (3) there should be no evidence of peri-splenic adhesions or scarring of the spleen; (4) the spleen should be normal on both gross inspection and histological examination. Crate et al. [11] added a fifth criterion which stated that result of serological examination should not show any significant rise in viral antibody titers that are suggestive of recent infection with viruses associated with splenic involvement.

Multiple Causative Factors

Various causative factors (table 1) have been implicated in non-traumatic pathological rupture of the spleen, most commonly being hematological malignancies [12], in which fragmentation and dissolution of the fibrous capsule of the spleen occur by infiltrating atypical lymphocytes, as seen in lymphoma/leukemia [13]. Malaria is the most common cause of pathologic rupture of spleen in the tropics, and life-threatening complications occur in up to an estimated 2% of patients [14]. Most cases of pathologic rupture of the spleen in malaria occur during acute infection, generally recognized within 3-4 days of the onset of symptoms viz. the primary attack [15] while chronically enlarged spleens are less vulnerable to rupture [13]. Spontaneous splenic rupture is more common with *P. vivax* than *Plasmodium falciparum* malaria.

Mechanism of Injury

Wiedemann first defined the term as resulting from an "incident without external force", NSR is a rare phenomenon in a histologically proven normal spleen, and in such cases, is called a spontaneous splenic rupture. Knoblich first distinguished the non-traumatic rupture of a pathological spleen from the extremely rare non-traumatic splenic rupture of unknown origin [16]. The proposed reason for the rupture is thought to be the size of the organ but normal-sized organs have also been reported with ruptured spleen [17].

Different mechanisms have been implicated in the process include elevated intra-splenic tension which is generally caused by cellular hyperplasia, compression by the abdominal musculature during physiological activities like sneezing, coughing and defecation and finally, vascular occlusion from reticular endothelial hyperplasia, which results in thrombosis and infarction. Infectious diseases especially mononucleosis, induce a swelling of the spleen due to hyperplasia of the pulpa and hyperaemia of the sinus and mantle plexus [18]. In malignant disorders the swelling of the spleen is caused by infiltrating malignant cells and extramedullary haematopoiesis [19]. This leads to interstitial and subcapsular hemorrhage and stripping of the capsule consequently further subcapsular aggravating the gross anatomic changes. [20, 21]

Table 1. Causative Factors of non-traumatic rupture of spleen

Condition	Disorders
Hematological	Coagulations disorders, leukemia, myelofibrosis, multiple myeloma
Metabolic Storage disease	Amyloidosis, Wilson's disease, Gaucher's disease
Infective	Bacterial: Staphylococcus, Streptococus, hemophilus Viral: CMV, VZ, HIV, dengue, infectious mononucleosis Protozoal: malaria, Kala-azar Others: Syphilis, hydatid disease
Drug Intake	Anticoagulation therapy, GCSF
Miscellaneous	Malignancy, splenic vein thrombosis, connective tissue disorders

Diagnosis: "Always Suspect!"

The management of non-traumatic or traumatic splenic hemorrhage has been a matter of debate constantly. The most common symptom of splenic rupture is left upper quadrant abdominal pain. This pain can become generalized, with distention, tenderness and rigidity as peritonitis sets in. Pallor, tachycardia, hypotension and oliguria may accompany the abdominal symptoms and eventually hemorrhagic shock if left untreated [8, 22]. Two other signs that are suggestive of splenic rupture are Kehr's sign (left diaphragmatic irritation resulting in referred pain to the left shoulder) and Balance's sign (palpable tender mass in the left upper quadrant). Diagnosis is based on clinical symptoms and relevant diagnostic tests. Radiological imaging can play an important role in diagnosing when a ruptured spleen is suspected. Plain abdominal radiographs can show enlargement of the spleen with medial displacement of the gastric bubble and elevation of the left hemidiaphragm with impaired motion. [23] Focused assessment with sonography for trauma (FAST) is an excellent modality to obtain a quick diagnosis of intra-peritoneal fluid [9]. This is a safe method to look for the presence of fluid in the peritoneal cavity. Although it is an operator-depended technique, it is still considered the best imaging method for the initial evaluation of unstable patients. The limitations of FAST are its inability to identify the type and source of the fluid and it may not detect fluid volumes less than 200 to 500 milliliters.

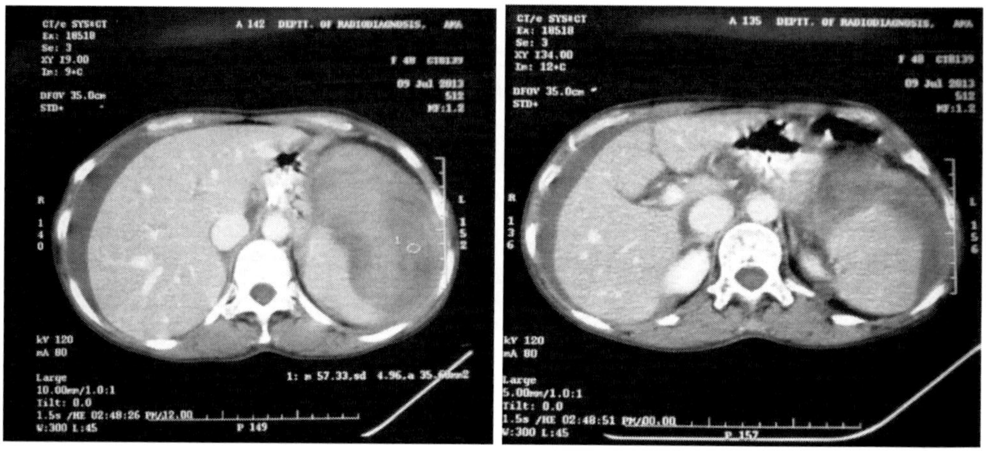

Figure 1. 38 yrs old lady with history of chronic cough and no trauma presented to surgical emergency with acute abdomen. CECT abdomen revealed Grade III splenic injury.

FAST can be combined with aspiration of the free fluid when the fluid is easy accessible to determine the type of fluid. Angiography though not in fashion, include extravasation of contrast, a "mottled" parenchymal phase and arteriovenous shunts with early venous filling and bowing, stretching and crowding of the vessels. [23] CT abdomen clearly shows grade of splenic damage severity and intraperitoneal free fluid but is reserved for stable patients [6]. CT has a sensitivity and specificity of at least 95% in detecting splenic injury. [24]

Management: "Less is Better Appraoch"

The English literature is ample with data supporting the role of non-operative management of traumatic low-grade splenic injuries in hemodynamically stable trauma patients same principle has been applied for the management of non-traumatic splenic rupture [28]. Aggressive management with early surgical intervention is important [25]. The survival of patients following splenectomy is probably well correlated with the course of the underlying disease. Of the 24 patients described since 1960 (including described above) 17 patients underwent splenectomy. Historically the treatment of choice for all kinds of splenic rupture used to be splenectomy; however, nowadays it remains subject to debate. Splenectomy remains the treatment of choice in patients with a hemoperitoneum and severe hypovolemic shock. During laparotomy repair of the spleen or tamponade by the use of an absorbable mesh (splenorraphy) should be considered to preserve splenic tissue. [26, 27]

Conservative management consists of observation for 7 to 14 days in the hospital, strict bed rest and administration of fluid and blood as needed.[29-30] Rupture usually occurs within the first week of illness, although it may happen in any time of the course of the disease (1-30 days).[29-30] An alternative to surgery is emergency transcatheter arterial embolisation, when patients are responsive to initial fluid resuscitation since preservation of viable splenic tissue is considered preferable. [32-34] There are some reports that indicate that spleen function remains even after embolisation of the proximal splenic artery due to collateral circulation. [35-37] With improved surgical techniques and supportive care, keeping in view the preoperative and post operative risk of splenectomy there has been an emergence of splenic conservation especially in malaria endemic areas. [28, 38] Splenectomy should therefore be reserved for those patients with severe rupture or those with severe rupture or those with continued and recurrent bleeding. [15]

To conclude the treatment of hemodynamic stable patients with non-traumatic splenic ruptures should be assessed individually with a low threshold for surgery or arterial embolization.

References

[1] Lai P. K. Infectious mononucleosis: recognition and management. *Hosp. Pract.,* 1977; 12: 47-52.

[2] Laseter T., McReynolds T. Spontaneous splenic rupture. *Mil. Med.,* 2004; 169: 673-674.

[3] Badenoch D. F., Maurice H. D., Gilmore O. J. Spontaneous rupture of a normal spleen. *J. R. Coll. Surg. Edinb.,* 1985; 30:326-327.

[4] Schnarkowski P., Brecht-Krauß D., Goldmann A., Friedrich J. M. Sonographischer Nachweis von Milzverletzungen nach stumpfem Bauchtrauma. *Ultraschall in Med.,* 1991;12:293–6.

[5] Hyun B. M., Varga C. F., Rubin R. J. Spontaneous and pathologic rupture of the spleen. *Arch. Surg.,* 1972;104:652–7.

[6] Torricelli P., Coriani C., Marchetti M., Rossi A., Manenti A. Spontaneous rupture of the spleen: report of two cases. *Abdom. Imaging,* 2001; 26: 290-293.

[7] Tu A. S., Tran M. H. T., Larsen C. R. Spontaneous splenic rupure: report of five cases and a review of the literature. *Emerg. Radiol.,* 1997; 4: 415-418.

[8] Denehy T., McGrath E. W., Breen J. L. Splenic torsion and rupture in pregnancy. *Obstet. Gynecol. Surv.,* 1988; 43: 123-131.

[9] Klinkert P., Kluit A. B., de Vries A. C., Puylaert J. B. Spontaneous rupture of the spleen: role of ultrasound in diagnosis, treatment, and monitoring. *Eur. J. Surg.,* 1999; 165: 712-713.

[10] Orloff M. J., Peksin G. W. Spontaneous rupture of the normal spleen; a surgical enigma. *Int. Abstr. Surg.,* 1958; 106: 1-11.

[11] Crate I. D., Payne M. J. Is the diagnosis of spontaneous rupture of a normal spleen valid? *J. R. Army Med. Corps.,* 1991; 137: 50-51.

[12] Oinonen R., Franssila K., Elonen E. Spontaneous splenic rupture in two patients with a blastoid variant of mantle cell lymphoma. *Ann. Hematol.,* 1997; 74: 33-35.

[13] Debnath D., Valerio D. Atraumatic rupture of the spleen in adults. *J. R. Coll. Surg. Edinb.,* 2002; 47: 437-445.

[14] Jimenez B. C., Navarro M., Huerga H., Lopez-Velez R. Spontaneous splenic rupture due to Plasmodium vivax in a traveler: case report and review. *J. Travel Med.,* 2007; 14: 188-191.

[15] Zingman B. S., Viner B. L. Splenic complications in malaria: case report and review. *Clin. Infect. Dis.*, 1993; 16: 223-232.

[16] Knoblich R. Pathologic (so-called spontaneous) rupture of the spleen in leukemia and lymphoma. *Mich. Med.*, 1966; 65:105–10.

[17] Zieren J., Paul M., Scharfenberg M., Muller J. M. The spontaneous splenic rupture as first manifestation of mantle cell lymphoma, a dangerous rarity. *Am. J. Emerg. Med.*, 2004; 22: 629-631.

[18] Mortelmans C., Populaire J. Spontaneous splenic rupture in infections mononucleosis. *Acta. Chir. Bel.*, 1993;93:193–5.

[19] Giagoundis A. A., Burk M., Meckenstock G., Kocht J., Schneider W. Pathologic rupture of the spleen in hematologic malignancies. *Ann. Haematol.*, 1996;73:297–302.

[20] Yagmur Y., Kara I. H., Aldemir M., Buyukbayram H., Tacyildiz I. H., Keles C. Spontaneous rupture of malarial spleen: two case reports and review of literature. *Crit. Care,* 2000; 4: 309-313.

[21] Patel M. I. Spontaneous rupture of a malarial spleen. *Med. J. Aust.*, 1993; 159: 836-837.

[22] Toubia N. T., Tawk M. M., Potts R. M., Kinasewitz G. T. Cough and spontaneous rupture of a normal spleen. *Chest,* 2005; 128: 1884-1886.

[23] Love L., Greenfield G. B., Braun T. W., Moncada R., Freeark R. J., Baker R. J. Angiography of splenic trauma. *Radiology,* 1968; 91(1):96-102.

[24] Jeffrey R. B., Laing F. C., Federle M. P., Goodman P. C. Computed tomography of splenic trauma. *Radiology,* 1981; 141(3):729-32.

[25] Bernat S., Garcia Boyero R., Guinot M., Lopez F., Gozalbo T., Canigral G. Pathologic rupture of the spleen as the initial manifestation in acute lymphoblastic leukemia. *Haematologica,* 1998; 83: 760-761.

[26] Hamel C. T., Blum J., Harder F., Kocher T. Nonoperative treatment of splenic rupture in malaria tropica: a review of literature and case report. *Acta Tropica*, 2002; 82(1):1-5.

[27] Leemans R., van Mourik J. B. A spleen-preserving method in splenic rupture using an absorbable net. *Ned. Tijdschr. Geneeskd.,* 1988; 132(44):2016-7.

[28] Brichkov I., Cummings L., Fazylov R., Horovitz J. H. Nonoperative management of spontaneous splenic rupture in infectious mononucleosis: the role for emerging diagnostic and treatment modalities. *Am. Surg.*, 2006; 72: 401-404.

[29] Körner M., Krötz M. M., Degenhart C., Pfeifer K. J., Reiser M. F., Linsenmaier U. Current Role of Emergency US in Patients with Major Trauma. *Radiographics, 2008;* 28(1):225-42.

[30] Julià J., Canet J. J., Lacasa X. M., González G., Garau J. Spontaneous spleen rupture during typhoid fever. *Int. J. Infect. Dis.,* 2000; 4(2):108-9.

[31] Lin W. C., Chen Y. F., Lin C. H., Tzeng Y. H., Chiang H. J., Ho Y. J., Shen W. C., Chen J. H. Emergent transcatheter arterial embolization in hemodynamically unstable patients with blunt splenic injury. *Acad. Radiol.,* 2008; 15(2):201-8.

[32] Wei B., Hemmila M. R., Arbabi S., Taheri P. A., Wahl W. L. Angioembolization reduces operative intervention for blunt splenic injury. *J. Trauma,* 2008; 64(6):1472-7.

[33] Lui B., Schlicht S., Vrazas J. Role of embolization in the management of splenic trauma. *Australas Radiol.,* 2004; 48(3):401-3.

[34] Bellingham G. A., Kribs S., Kornecki A., Scott L., Leaker M., Fraser D. D. Proximal splenic artery embolization in the management of splenic rupture. *Pediatr. Crit. Care Med.*, 2009; 10(1):e1-4.

[35] Loffroy R., Guiu B., Cercueil J. P., Lepage C., Cheynel N., Steinmetz E., Ricolfi F., Krausé D. Transcatheter arterial embolization of splenic artery aneurysms and pseudoaneurysms: short- and long-term results. *Ann. Vasc. Surg.,* 2008; 22(5):618-26.

[36] Laganà D., Carrafiello G., Mangini M., Fontana F., Dizonno M., Castelli P, Fugazzola C. Endovascular treatment of splenic artery aneurysms. *Radiol. Med.,* 2005; 110(1-2): 77-87.

[37] Shaw J. H. F., Print C. G.: Postsplenectomy sepsis. *Br. J. Surg.,* 1989, 76: 1074 –1081.

[38] Mokashi A. J., Shirahatti R. G., Prabhu S. K., Vagholkar K. R.: Pathological rupture of malarial spleen. *J. Postgrad. Med.,* 1992; 38:141–142.

In: Rare Diseases
Editors: Giorgio Di Giovanni and Pietro Marcoz

ISBN: 978-1-62948-525-6

Chapter X

DevelopAKUre: Curing the World's First Genetic Disease

Oliver Timmis*
Head of Projects, AKU Society, UK

Abstract

Alkaptonuria (AKU) is the world's first genetic disease. Discovered over 100 years ago, it still has no cure. For the past decade, the AKU Society has worked towards patients' dreams of finding an effective treatment. Through funding basic research, building clinical knowledge of AKU and collaborating with industry and clinical trial experts, the AKU Society is close to achieving this. We united our contacts into a public-private partnership, called the DevelopAKUre consortium. Together we raised €6 million through a European Commission Seventh Framework Programme grant with a further €4 million through co-financing.

After seeking scientific advice from the European Medicines Agency (EMA), we launched a series of international clinical trials in November last year. They incorporate three studies: SONIA 1 (a phase II dose-ranging study), SONIA 2 (a phase III clinical efficacy study) and SOFIA (a comparison study of young and old AKU patients to assess what age is best to begin treatment).

The AKU Society is leading on patient recruitment and retention and has faced many challenges converting our experiences of recruitment in the UK for a national treatment centre into recruitment throughout Europe for clinical trials. In this article, we discuss the difficulties in diagnosis of a rare disease, the lessons learnt from building an international consortium to launch clinical trials and the challenges in running patient recruitment on a European scale.

* E-mail: oliver.

Introduction

Alkaptonuria (AKU) is the world's first genetic disease. Discovered over 100 years ago, by Sir Archibald Garrod, it still has no cure. The DevelopAKUre project aims to change this through a series of clinical trials to determine the effectiveness of a new treatment: a drug called nitisinone. DevelopAKUre is unique: it is a patient-centric programme working in a public-private partnership to try to cure a rare disease. We hope that our experiences could lead to a new model for clinical research, a model that embraces the need for clinical, regulatory and academic knowledge alongside the expertise from patients.

The AKU Society is a charity founded to support patients with AKU and ultimately to find a cure. We knew that this would be impossible by ourselves, so gradually we have built contacts in academia and industry to help us.

The AKU Society funded the creation of animal and cell models at the University of Liverpool, which have shown a reduction of alkaptonuric disease after treatment with nitisinone [1]. Additionally, our collaboration at the Royal Liverpool University Hospital led to a quantitative AKU severity score index [2], which is now used as one of the secondary endpoints in the AKU clinical trials.

AKU is an ultra-orphan disease, affecting around 1 in 500,000 in Europe, which means there are few patients with the disease. An ongoing goal for the AKU Society is to find these patients, to offer them support, advice and, now, to inform them of clinical research. In the UK, our patient identification campaigns focused on General Practitioners (GPs). In fact, the majority of UK patients we know were found through a mail campaign to over 11,000 UK GP practices [3]. However, our ultimate aim remained to find a treatment for AKU. Our best option is an ex-weedkiller, a drug called nitisinone (see Figure 1). Nitisinone is approved for the treatment of a related condition, hereditary tyrosinaemia type I. As both diseases use the same biochemical pathway, there is good evidence that the same drug should work. The US National Institutes of Health (NIH) began trials of the drug in AKU patients, yet never collected sufficient evidence to decide on its effectiveness [4]. For the past decade, the AKU Society has aimed to complete these trials to decide conclusively if nitisinone could treat AKU.

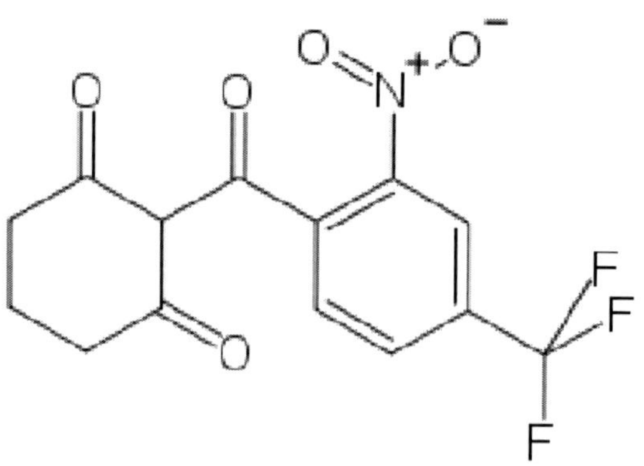

Figure 1. Chemical structure of nitisinone (marketed by Sobi as Orfadin®). IUPAC name: 2-[2-nitro-4-(trifluoromethyl)benzoyl]cyclohexane-1,3-dione.

Building a Consortium

To complete clinical trials in a rare disease, we would require a consortium of partners. The members of the DevelopAKUre consortium are listed in Table 1, which shows how we brought together companies with different backgrounds. The coordinating partner is the lead clinical centre – the Royal Liverpool University Hospital – headed by our Primary Investigator, Prof L Ranganath. The trials are sponsored by the University of Liverpool, meaning they are legally responsible for the wellbeing of patients, the insurance of the trial and the accuracy of all results.

For a rare disease, it is vital to spread recruitment as widely as possible – that is why we included partners in France and Slovakia. With three trial centres covering large parts of Europe, we can contact a much greater number of patients. Where available, each clinical centre is supported by a patient group. We handle recruitment in the UK and parts of Europe not covered by a clinical centre. In France, our sister group, ALCAP, as well as the Institut Necker, will help with the patient recruitment and travel. There is no group in Slovakia, something that we are trying to address by launching an AKU Society Slovakia this year.

Table 1. Members of the DevelopAKUre consortium

	Partner Name	Country	Main Role in DevelopAKUre
Hospitals	Royal Liverpool University Hospital	UK	Clinical trial centre in the UK (Co-ordinator)
	National Institute of Rheumatic Disease	Slovakia	Clinical trial centre in Slovakia
	Assistance Publique Hopitaux de Paris	France	Clinical trial centre in France
Patient Groups	AKU Society	UK	Patient recruitment, patient support and dissemination for Europe
	ALCAP	France	Patient recruitment, patient support and dissemination for France and Belgium
Universities	University of Liverpool	UK	Data analysis, ear cartilage biopsy As sponsor: insurance of trials, wellbeing of patients, accuracy of results
	University of Siena	Italy	Data analysis
	Institute of Molecular Physiology and Genetics	Slovakia	Genetic analysis
Others	PSR Group	Netherlands	Clinical trial monitors, data recording
	Cudos	Netherlands	Protocol writing
	Nordic Bioscience	Denmark	Biomarker analysis
	Sobi	Sweden	Drug supply and regulatory support
	Institut Necker	France	Patient recruitment, refunding patient costs

We have found that often the best way to find and help patients is by using local knowledge (patients and doctors) to build patient groups. Usually patients prefer hearing from people who can relate to their disease and so patient groups can help give credibility to a recruitment campaign.

The universities and SMEs (Small-Medium Enterprises) are important for the analysis of clinical data. Our studies will collect genetic material to be analysed in Slovakia, human tissues to be examined by Liverpool and biomarker analysis will be completed in Italy and Denmark.

Among the most crucial partners are a CRO (Contract Research Organisation) and consultancy, PSR Group and Cudos, which are writing the trial protocols, clinical handbooks and monitoring the clinical research to ensure it is done to the highest possible standard. This is to guarantee that the results are reliable and accurate. Finally, we have Sobi, a pharmaceutical company that owns the drug. They will be providing the drug to all study sites, giving advice on the trials and most importantly, providing regulatory advice. The main aim of the studies, if we prove nitisinone is a useful treatment, is to gain approval for its use. Sobi will then lead on a Marketing Authorisation Application to the European Medicines Agency (EMA) which, if successful, would license the drug for use in treating all European AKU patients.

Funding

To fund the newly developed consortium, we applied to the European Commission's Seventh Framework Programme (FP7) under their call: Pre-clinical and Clinical Research for Rare Diseases. The grant of €6 million would just barely cover the costs of the clinical programme we had devised. The application was successful, enabling us to launch the DevelopAKUre project on 1 November 2012.

As the goal of the project is to apply for marketing authorisation, we went to the EMA for advice on the studies. Together, we created DevelopAKUre as a series of three connected clinical research studies, listed in Table 2. Starting in early 2013, we began a dose-ranging trial called SONIA 1. This is due to finish this summer, before the 4-year study, SONIA 2 starts at the end of 2013. Alongside SONIA 2, we will run SOFIA – a cross-sectional study to better understand how AKU develops and at what age is the optimum time to begin treatment.

Table 2. The three parts of DevelopAKUre

Trial Name	Description	Sites
SONIA 1: Suitability Of Nitisinone In Alkaptonuria 1	3-month phase II study for safety and dose-ranging.	UK/Slovakia
SONIA 2: Suitability Of Nitisinone In Alkaptonuria 2	4-year phase III clinical effectiveness study to compare nitisinone to a non-treatment group to determine effectiveness.	UK/Slovakia/ France
SOFIA: Subclinical Ochronosis Features In Alkaptonuria	Cross-sectional study to compare young/old AKU patients to determine age to start treatment.	UK

Challenges

The main issue in DevelopAKUre – as with all clinical trials focusing on a rare disease – has been patient recruitment. We have estimated around 500 patients in Europe (see Figure 2) – taken from our patient identification campaigns. For statistically significant research we need at least 140 AKU patients in our phase III trial. Removing children and the elderly from the identified number means that we need to recruit nearly all available patients in Europe. That is not an easy task and one that we are still trying to complete.

Our best method of patient recruitment has been to work through local AKU Societies we have helped to create. However, in Europe the problem is compounded by language barriers. The main European languages (English, French, Germany, Italian and Spanish) still only cover a small proportion of people, and therefore to contact every patient is difficult. Our trial website (available at www.developAKUre.eu) contains those five languages as well as Dutch and Slovak to represent the members of our consortium. Again, to spread the message more widely, we have relied on local knowledge. We are fortunate that many AKU patients in Europe are multi-lingual and so speak at least one of the languages we use. However, we know that it means we are still unable to contact or even communicate with all AKU patients.

Another potential problem was having patient groups (the AKU Society and ALCAP) working together in a consortium with a pharmaceutical company (Sobi). Interactions between these types of groups are heavily regulated, especially in the UK, where the ABPI (The Association of The British Pharmaceutical Industry) has produced codes of practise to ensure that the pharmaceutical industry and patient groups can work together without undue interference.

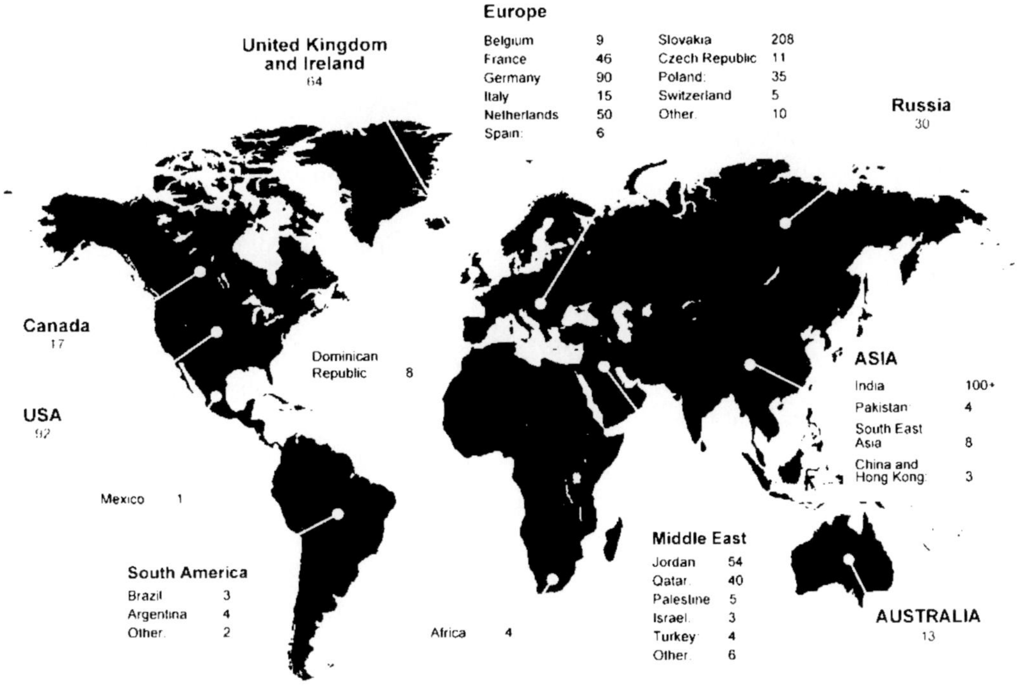

Figure 2. AKU Patient Identification around the World.

Our relationship with Sobi has worked well: the funding is transparent through a grant from the European Commission, and we are all dedicated to the same goal. Nitisinone has been linked with a treatment for AKU for many years, and regardless of the outcome of the trials, we can finally answer the question of its effectiveness. We have shown that it is relatively easy to overcome the potential difficulties by remembering that the ultimate aim for all parties is the patients' benefit.

Conclusion

DevelopAKUre is unique: it is an example of clinical research where patient groups have been involved from the start. We funded basic research and observational studies to learn about AKU. With this knowledge, we could test a new treatment, nitisinone, in a mouse model. We helped build a consortium, with the expertise to plan and run clinical trials of nitisinone. We gathered funding from the European Commission, and now are finding and recruiting patients to take part in research. We are still a few years off the end of DevelopAKUre and finding out whether the drug is capable of treating the disease, but we hope that our journey so far gives hope for a new idea in clinical research. The main conclusion is that patients should be involved with research into their own disease. We hope to encourage patient groups to take control of their clinical research and to give credence to pharmaceutical companies wishing to engage with patients.

For further information on the AKU clinical trials, please see the trial website; available at: www.developAKUre.eu.

References

[1] Preston A. J., Keenan C. M., Sutherland H., et al. Ochronotic arthropathy in a mouse model of alkaptonuria and its inhibition by nitisinone. *Ann. Rheum. Dis.,* 2013 Mar. 19 [Epub ahead of print].

[2] Cox T. F., Ranganath L. A. quantitative assessment of alkaptonuria: testing the reliability of two disease severity scoring systems. *J. Inherit. Metab. Dis.,* 2011 Dec; 34 (6): 1153-62.

[3] Ranganath L., Taylor A. M., Shenkin A., et al. Identification of alkaptonuria in the general population: a United Kingdom experience describing the challenges, possible solutions and persistent barriers. *J. Inherit. Metab. Dis.,* 2011 Jun;34 (3): 723-30.

[4] Introne W. J., Perry M. B., Troendle J., et al. A 3 year randomized therapeutic trial of nitisinone in alkaptonuria. Introne WJ et al. *Mol. Genet. Metab.,* 2011 Aug; 103 (4):307-14.

Index

D

E

F

G

H

I

J

K

L

M

Q

R

S

T

U